To Cure and to Care

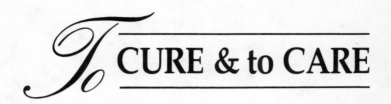

To CURE & to CARE

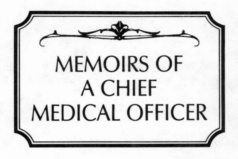

MEMOIRS OF
A CHIEF
MEDICAL OFFICER

James Deeny

THE GLENDALE PRESS

First published in Ireland by
THE GLENDALE PRESS LTD.
18 Sharavogue
Glenageary Road Upper
Dun Laoghaire
Co. Dublin, Ireland.

British Library Cataloguing in Publication Data

Deeny, James, *1906-*
To cure and to care: memoirs of a chief medical officer
1.   Ireland. Medicine. Deeny, James, *1906-*
I.   Title
610'.92'4

ISBN 0-907606-64-4
ISBN 0-907606-62-8 pbk

Cover by David L. Murphy
Typeset by Wendy A. Commins, The Curragh
Make-up by Paul Bray Studio
Printed by The Guernsey Press Co. Ltd.,
Channel Islands.

To Gemma, who chose the title for this book,
for more than 50 years of love and companionship.
And to Michael, Gillian, Tressan and James
who joined us on the way

To the 'backroom' men and women in the
health professions everywhere, who create
health services, promote health and save lives

Ut Sciat ut sciatur scire ut doceat

St Augustine. *Motives of Learning*

'A constituent man,' said the Sergeant, 'largely instrumental but volubly fervous.'

Flan O'Brien. *The Third Policeman*

Be supple in things immaterial

R.L. Stevenson. *Kidnapped*

The peace of all things is the tranquillity of order.

St Augustine. *The City of God*

Though our songs cannot banish ancient wrongs,
Though they follow where the rose goes,
And their sound swooning over the hollow ground,
Fades and leaves the enchanted air, bare.

Yet the wise say that not unblest he dies,
Who has known a single May day.
If we have laughed, loved and
Laboured in our craft, we may pass with a resigned mind.

Walter Raleigh (Trans.). Old Gaelic court poem

Contents

Introduction

I n recent times, health systems in countries world-wide are the subject of unprecedented change. At one end of a scale, successful developments and progress are being achieved by the implementation of the concept *Health for All by the Year 2000*, the Declaration of the WHO International Conference on Primary Health Care at Alma-Ata, USSR, in 1978. At the other end, in many countries, social control of health systems through politics, economics, administration or ethics is bringing about very large and possibly regressive changes. Whether due to financial cuts, the introduction of new management personnel and techniques, attempted changes in purpose, the distribution of resources, or changes in structures and functions, health systems are being altered very considerably.

For the professionals engaged in the health systems of many advanced countries, that is, the doctors, nurses, bio-medical scientists and technologists and all the others either concerned with the laying on of hands on sick people or in front-line support, the present situation creates confusion, unhappiness and doubt. As a great Swedish doctor said recently 'the ascent of Swedish medicine has been generated by the doctors while the descent is now headed by the administrators'. There is an unhappy conflict and the public suffer.

The raw material of a health system is man and there is more to man in relation to the health system than science, politics, economics, bureaucracy and all the rest of it. We are moving away from the basic essential of any health system which is Care. As Father Henri Nouwen of Yale says 'What we see and like to see is cure and change. But what we do not see and do not want to see is Care, the participation in the pain, the solidarity in suffering, the sharing in the experience of brokenness. And still, cure without care is as dehumanising as a gift given with a cold heart.'

We might think of any national health system as an evolving thing, with the participation of a great number of people contributing through their ideas, inventions, hard work and intelligence to its evolution. This stream is moved through the genius of researchers, by changes in cultures, by prosperity or adversity, by centres of excellence, by the international exchange of ideas and by all kinds of things. The stream changes course from time to time, as one group of ideas is challenged by another. From the resulting conflict comes a synthesis or compromise or superlative. When a synthesis is reached another thesis or proposition is produced and the change and movement starts up all over again.

The health professionals have to come to terms with social control. They cannot, however, be pushed into a corner. Their knowledge, expertise, experience and judgement must be appreciated. Administrators, while an essential part, must realise that they cannot run a health system from their offices. In fact it is almost a maxim in WHO, that when a technically sound project fails it is due to faulty administration. Health systems have two components, social and economic. If economists take over and stress too much the economic aspects they can damage the social component. Politicians are important. As the elected representatives of the people they must lead. It is their job to introduce effective legislation, deal fairly with the conflicting interests in democracy, handle difficult situations wisely and provide a leadership for all the elements in the health system. They should operate, without too much egoism, an honest 'feed-back' system to inform the public. Politicians must be measured against such standards.

I have spent sixty years of a professional life in this debate ranging from the level of private practitioner in a small town in the North of Ireland through the national to the international level in various fields. I present my professional autobiography as a sort of case study, of what it was like to be a member of that endangered species and indeed possibly dying breed of Chief Medical Adviser, Chief Medical Officer, Director of Health Services, Health Commissioner, Vice-Minister of Health or whatever the title. I have been a 'Chief' for twenty-five years or so and one of the brethren, but their day seems to be over. In Sweden for the first time in three hundred years the top administrator of the Swedish Board of Health is no longer a doctor. In the NHS in England, one of the supremos was a supermarket executive. In many countries, administrators who see life through the medium of files, or accountants who count costs are in control or politicians, influenced by controversial ideologies or party hang-ups.

I started medicine in the pre-antibiotic days sixty years ago and my training was a mixture of the old Victorian type of clinical practice and the beginning of scientific medicine as we know it. I experienced the working life of a practitioner in the Hungry Thirties in a poverty-stricken linen town in the North of Ireland. Later I was one of the team which over a period of twenty years, working from the Department of Health in the Custom House, created a modern health service in the Republic of Ireland. During twenty years our team played a great part in bringing down the annual toll of 4,175 deaths of infants under one year who died in 1941, to 1,827 in 1961 and laid a foundation for the decline which has our present figure amongst the best in the world. People between the age of five years and fifty-five who died in Ireland in 1941 numbered 9,277; by 1961 we had this figure reduced to 2,838. Everyone dies sooner or later, but we enabled a lot of people to live longer or at least to avoid an early death.

The story goes further. First, I experienced international medicine in Third World field projects starting in 1956 and then as Chief of Mission for the World Health Organisation in Indonesia. After other tasks for WHO such as training the first group of people to come from the USSR to work with WHO, I became the first Chief of Senior Staff Training in Geneva, which involved setting up and directing the programmes of training, recycling and development of the senior staff of the World Health Organisation. When I retired, I became Scientific Adviser in the Vatican and later took up other occupations before settling down to farm here in Rosslare in County Wexford, Ireland.

I moved along through the stream at different levels over the sixty years and it seems important in the present day whirl of events that some human aspects should be considered.

So I began this book four years ago. I wrote it out in longhand and when I had said all I had to say, my nephew Arthur

Deeny, typed it out for me and started the tidying up of my 600 pages of script. It was read by Tom Barrington, Des Roche, J.B. Lyons and John O'Connell, friends of mine who I trusted to treat it gently and yet be sufficiently honest in their comments. I had encouragement in the beginning to undertake the job from Denis MacClean. I would like to acknowledge the help I received from Dr Ruth Barrington, an amiable young lady of intelligence whose admirable book, *Health Medicine and Politics in Ireland 1900-1970*, is well-researched and conclusive. In the end I bought a Wang word processor, taught myself to use it and produced various renderings until the final version was reached. Tony Farmar edited it, cut it in half, tidied it up and thanks to Microdot, made the manuscript presentable for my publisher, Tom Turley of Glendale Press, to whom I am indebted for his kindness and patience. After all, when you get to 81 years, you need a bit of help.

1

Practice in Lurgan

N O ONE wants to hear of my growing up in Lurgan, of my family history or of my schooling so I shall start my story in 1931 when, after seven years of medical training, I underwent that important 'rite of passage' for a young doctor sixty years ago and 'put up my plate'. This was in Church Place, Lurgan in September 1931. Lurgan was a linen-manufacturing town of sixteen thousand people in County Armagh, Northern Ireland. It was the world-centre for the manufacture of linen handkerchiefs, but it had no other particular claim to distinction. It was situated in a pleasant countryside and was near to Lough Neagh, the largest lake in these islands. The people of the town and surrounding districts were almost equally divided into two factions which denoted their religious, political, cultural, economic and social characteristics. The members of the two factions rarely mixed. The people of both factions were the salt of the earth.

Putting up the plate might simply be regarded as screwing a brass plate with your name on it on to the wall or on the door of the premises in which you started practice. But it was really very much more. For the young doctor, finished with his hospital service and deciding to go into general practice, it meant selecting the district or area where you would settle down. This depended on 'openings', such as some older practitioner dying, service in a local hospital, your hopes of securing patients because of your family background or your sporting ability or anything else which might recommend you to the public and enable you to get started.

There were dispensary doctor appointments but these were generally to be got only by political influence and in the North of Ireland, Catholic doctors did not have much chance of such posts or of appointments to the local hospitals. You also looked for a house which provided a 'good stand' and which you could afford, usually to rent, since very few people putting up a plate had much capital and your savings had to last you till you started to make a bit of money.

Then there was the question of furnishing the place, a 'surgery' and waiting room and some sort of living accommodation, since all doctors lived over the shop. A housekeeper was necessary, not only to look after the place and answer the door to patients but to cook and wash for you. Later one had to have a car. There were exciting things like having a wash-basin put into the surgery, equipping yourself with some instruments, and putting your few books into a book-case to make an impression of learning and scholarship. If you were going to dispense, then you laid in some 'stock' mixtures which you would dilute to make up cough bottles, digitalis for heart disease, antacids for stomach troubles and so on. You had 'Tabloid Products B. W. & Co' for injection and splints and bandages and things like needles and sutures for sewing up cuts. There was a lot of thought given to fitting out the midwifery bag. Of course the representatives of the drug houses laid siege to you, looking for orders.

It was usually great fun, but there was equally a great strain in that you were gambling your whole future on your success. However, once you had screwed the plate to the door you were in business. That done you had to show yourself around. You drove, cycled or walked around the town, trying to look very busy as if you were rushing to patients here and there. You called on people like the clergy to make yourself known, in the hope that they would tell their 'hearers' that you were a nice young man and a good doctor. You could attend the local dances, or if a Protestant join an Orange Lodge, play rugby for the local team and in every way get sufficient local notoriety to become known.

You took your courage in your hands and called on the other doctors, who felt that you were coming to take away their practices and you knew that you were but wanted them to know that you would do it nicely and painlessly.

You opened a bank account and you resisted insurance agents and encyclopaedia salesmen and a multitude of others who came to sell you something. Most young doctors were sitting ducks for a gentle 'rip off' as they had absolutely no business sense. Whether you were conscious of it or not, you became immediately a great item of gossip in the small town or district that you had selected in which to pitch your tent. Every young woman in the area sized you up, was 'dying to meet you', perhaps ruled you out as husband material, or perhaps considered you were worth a try.

The main thing was to keep busy or at least to seem busy. My mother told me that shortly after her marriage to my father, who went through this 'rite of passage' as a young doctor in Lurgan, she had remarked to him that compared to the number of people coming to the door, there was very little money to show for all the traffic. My father explained that it was important to create confidence and that there should be seen to be a lot of such activity. He created this by asking people to send up samples of urine or to send up for medicine or to send messages on how the patient felt or anything else he could think of. The main point was to bring them to his door and to get them accustomed to coming.

The first patients were mostly the local hypochondriacs, 'trying' the new doctor. In any community, no matter how well served by the existing medical practitioners, there are always cases which have been missed. In addition there are always people who have persistent complaints for which the existing men have had no cures. The new doctor, by finding a new dimension, might cure the odd one. The word is spread around that the 'new man' is good, and so it goes on. In such a way some of the greatest doctors in past generations have got their start.

I had some of this excitement but missed a lot of the rest of the fun because I simply moved next door to my father's practice. Although I had managed a good honours in the Final examination in Queen's University, I was not offered a job as house surgeon, since the Royal Victoria Hospital seldom appointed Catholics. In those days, in that vast hospital there was not a single Catholic medical on the staff. This does not mean that I was not well taught or treated as a student, or that I was not awarded an honour if I had earned it, or that I did not make good friends, but in the North the system was the system. However it did not worry me very much as I was needed at home. My father had a very large practice and was seriously overworked.

In those days the vast majority of practices were single-handed or doctors were often assisted by their sons. With his usual foresight, my father had sent me back to Queen's to do a BSc in biochemistry, bacteriology and pathology and, to make sure I was not idle, entered me for the two-year course for the Diploma in Public Health. I got the BSc and the first half of the DPH the first year and in the next, finished it and had a shot at my MD. I did the Doctorate by the more difficult examination route. This put you at the mercy of the examiners, who could ask you anything that they could think up, whereas if you offered a thesis, they were on your ground. Anyway, they failed me.

I stayed at home while going through all this, travelling up and down by train the twenty miles from Lurgan to Belfast and in the evening helping with the surgery sessions, doing any maternity cases that my father was prepared to trust me with. At the week-ends, I was especially useful. This programme was pretty tough, but my mother and father both worked so hard themselves that they did not seem to think it was unusual. For the second attempt at the MD I went into digs in Belfast for three months and worked really hard and got it.

When I had finished the MD, I went down to Dublin and sat the two parts of the membership examination of the Royal College of Physicians together and passed. So by the time I was twenty-four, I had a Public Health Diploma, an MD with pathology as my subject as well as the membership of the Royal College of Physicians in General Medicine. I had also the BSc in bacteriology, biochemistry and pathology. I was full of science and academic nonsense. I was also completely immature and really hadn't a clue. However, I was serving my apprenticeship to my father, and with his guidance and surveillance and by working with the Lurgan people, in about ten years or so I really felt that maybe I would become a 'good' doctor.

My plate had to be different — not for me the usual brass effect. I got myself a bronze plate with my name in white enamel and put up some of the degrees after my name. I went further and had writing paper with my name and all the degrees at the top; my prescription sheets were similarly adorned. My father took a poor view of this nonsense, said that I was advertising, and if I was so fond of them I should have the degrees embroidered on my pyjamas.

In his day my father had been a very bright student and had originally thought of becoming a specialist surgeon and to this end had taken the Primary Fellowship examination of the Royal College of Surgeons. Because there were a lot of brothers and sisters to be educated, my grandfather Deeny felt that he should settle down and make a living, so he came to Lurgan and put up his plate, started practice and never sat his final Fellowship Examination.

When he saw me flaunting this academic nonsense about, he became irritated and he got my sister to give him a grind to bring him up-to-date, though he had always read his medical journals. Soon he felt confident and had a shot at the Final FRCSI. They failed him. But he went to Dublin, stayed out in Dun Laoghaire and worked and studied very hard for a few months and this time got it. So FRCSI went up on his plate.

There was more to it than just being mildly jealous of me. He had one of the largest practices in the North and was very well-thought-of, in particular he had a special interest in vaccines, which was widely known. People came for this treatment from far and near, but he always resented, as I did, that he had not been offered a hospital appointment because Catholics seldom got such things. So there was an element of proving something.

On my return from Dublin the gentleman who lived next door asked me in and said that he was giving up the house and asked did I want it. There and then I decided to have my own establishment.

About eighty years before, my great-grandfather had built a row of large Victorian-style houses. His son, my grandfather, lived in the first with his family which had originally included my mother. Father and mother had the next house where my sister, brother and I were reared and where my father had his practice. I took up residence in the third.

My father's practice was mixed. He had first a large industrial practice of factory workers and their families. This included all or almost all the Catholics and quite a large share of working-class Protestants. Then he had a great number of farmers, some of whom came from up to twenty miles away. The farmers liked him as he was 'country-minded', had grazing land on the shores of Lough Neagh and loved cattle. Then there was the usual mixed, middle-class, town element, most of whom were Protestants. He had three surgery sessions a day and mostly worked a twelve hour day. There were no half-holidays and he was lucky to get Sunday afternoon to himself.

He did a lot of widwifery. How much I cannot remember. When I was at my peak later, I averaged a little more than three hundred cases a year and he certainly did more than me. They were all home deliveries, at which he was very skilful. I often drove him on night calls when I was a student and I have seen him do five home deliveries in one night. My own maximum was three.

Sixty years ago, before things changed, general practice was much more interesting than now. As there were no antibiotics, practice included a very large element of abcesses, pleurisies, chronic bone disease and septic infections, which if not well treated could be fatal. There seem to have been more fractures; more people rode bicycles, there were always accidents with horses, the roads and footpaths were not so well paved and people seemed to fall about a lot. Most fractures were 'set' by the family doctor and people like my father had wonderful hands and a feel for bones and were really expert as 'bone-setters'.

You were always on the look-out for fevers such as typhoid and an epidemic of measles meant a lot of very sick children and some deaths. Acute pneumonias often struck people suddenly; they gasped for breath for days, bringing up large quantities of 'rusty' sputum and trying to hold on till the crisis occurred and then suddenly recovered. Sometimes when I was a student and people were very ill with pneumonia, I might be pulled out of my bed by my father to go and sit with them all night, sponging them, poulticing their lungs and helping them to clear their airways or giving them oxygen from a cylinder requisitioned from a welding plant in a garage. There was always the risk of missing an acute abdomen, perhaps a perforated duodenal ulcer or an appendicitis; in those days an hour or so made all the difference and without an operation there was the risk of peritonitis and death. The main thing about medicine then was that you did things yourself and were probably more close to the patient. Fewer people went to hospital and there were none of the wonder drugs that we have to-day.

By the time I had finished my degrees, my sister Sheelagh had qualified and was on hand to help my father, so that I could be spared. I had saved a little, so in 1930 I took myself off to Vienna. On the plane were two senior American doctors and we got into conversation. They were friendly and they brought me to the American Medical Association of Vienna and made me a member. I wanted to study the bacteriology of tuberculosis and with the help of the AMA I ended up in the State Serum Institute working under Loewenstein. He had just perfected the best-ever medium for growing the tubercle bacillus. But he had become the centre of a controversy, as he claimed to be able to culture the tubercle bacillus from the blood of people suffering from a great variety of diseases hitherto unconnected with tuberculosis. Few people believed him and bloods were sent to the laboratory from all over the world. Working with a Viennese medical student called Poldi Gerzner, it was our job for part of my time to culture these bloods.

It was suspected in the end that one of Loewenstein's technicians who was believed to suffer from tuberculosis had in some way contaminated the culture plates. I picked up a lot of information about the bacteriology of tuberculosis and learnt how to make Loewenstein's medium properly. I also enjoyed myself thoroughly doing things like swimming in the Danube, drinking the new wine at the heuriger farmhouses in the Wiener Wald and listening to the never-ending Strauss waltzes while I danced the night away. I had a trip to Budapest and took in the Salzburg Opera Festival and generally had such a good time that after six months I was broke and had to come home.

With the advent of the Stormont government and a gradually increasing recession, the administrators were finding the health services increasingly expensive and difficult to run. As the 1929 recession grew worse we had a very great increase in sickness. Tangible diseases such as tuberculosis, anaemia, rheumatic fever and so on grew in numbers and so did intangible conditions such as nervous diseases, depressions and anxiety. The whole community began to suffer from the malaise. Men hung around the street corners, looking hopeless, while their wives were under a terrible strain to keep the homes going and to feed the children on the miserable dole payments available at that time. There were no children's allowances, and in Belfast, the hypocritical members of the Board of Guardians cut down the Outdoor Relief allowances to such an extent that there were food riots.

When people are unemployed and in addition are under-nourished they do not feel well. If they have access to a free medical service they use it and the costs go up.[1] It was mainly the Catholics who were unemployed and so the costs of our panel or the government part of our practice soared. The Stormont administrators in their wisdom had assumed that costs should be the same per head for rich and poor districts and towns. Ours were of course very much above average.

So they started a rather nasty process which I can only describe as harassment as the administrators reacted to what they thought of as our extravagance. On one occasion my father and I were both fined £150 for over-prescribing. It was bad enough to feel that as Catholics you were second-class citizens and without redress, but to have it going on all the time was worrying. This was one reason why at fifty four years

1. The Panel System of Medical Care was introduced into Northern Ireland in or around 1930. It provided free medical care for all persons engaged in employment which was covered by insurance schemes operated by the Ministry of Labour. Men and women qualified by a number of stamps on an insurance card representing weeks worked, received free medical care, medicines, hospital and specialist treatment. People entitled, signed on 'the panel' of a doctor of their choice. My father and I had more than 7,000 people on our panel. Such treatment was not available under the scheme for their dependants. In the event of long-term unemployment, benefit lapsed. With unemployment there was an increased demand for health care. The Ministry of Labour studied the average cost per prescription and also per person treated and the frequency of the medical prescriptions. The cost of medicines for each practice was compared with the national 'norm'. Naturally practices in unemployment 'black-spots' cost more than in other areas. An attempt was made to control costs by penalising doctors who were 'over-prescribing'. Doctors were paid on a capitation basis.

of age, my father crucified himself for nearly a year taking one of the toughest exams there is, just to get a piece of paper certifying that he was a Fellow of the Royal College of Surgeons.

One of the interesting things I remember about our practice was our Sunday morning clinics. These were special sessions when we brought back cases which were of special interest and had a second look at them. Sometimes we could not make an immediate diagnosis and needed to do tests. When I was working in the laboratory at Queen's, I could bring up blood specimens for example and do a blood urea or a blood sugar test or the sort of simple check we did in those days.[2] It was a good opportunity to try out the kind of thing I was learning and anyway helped the patients. In addition I did test-meals, passing a fine tube down into people's stomachs to find out what was happening there by analysing the contents.[3] I also used a microscope I had, and did blood and sputum tests. In Queen's I made vaccines for my father's cases.

An example of the kind of thing we did was our study of the 'laudanum drinkers'. These were poor unfortunates, usually dreadfully anaemic, for whom my father prescribed a pint of laudanum, that is tincture of opium, each month. Some of these he had inherited from other doctors and some he had started off himself. The reason for the laudanum was that they had all chronic diarrhoea and laudanum was the only thing that could control it. Some were very 'dottery' and they were

2. The level of urea in the blood is a valuable indicator of kidney function. It is disturbed in cases of glomerular filtration in kidney failure and disease. Diabetes Mellitus is the name given to a range of metabolic disorders having in common an increase in the level of sugar in the blood and is usually accompanied by the excretion of sugar in the urine. The blood sugar test estimates the level of sugar in the blood.
3. Carbohydrate Fractional Test Meal is a simple method of investigating certain stomach functions. A slender rubber tube (Ryles) is passed into the stomach of a fasting patient, the resting contents are drawn off and measured and a simple test meal is then given. Samples are drawn off every 15 minutes until digestion is completed. Estimates are made of acidity, starch, blood (if any), resting acid and so on as well as the emptying time of the stomach. This technique, possibly a bit old fashioned to-day, was of great diagnostic value.

so uncoordinated in their gait that they could hardly walk
without falling all over the place.

In 1929 or 1930, Professor Sir W.W.D. Thompson of
Queen's brought his friend Sir Arthur Hurst over to Belfast to
lecture. He told us about his new discovery of spasm of the
end of the oesophagus or gullet and how to treat it. He touched
on the fact that people with pernicious anaemia were found
to have a lack of hydrochloric acid in their stomach secretions.
This was before the great Harvard discovery by Minot and
Murphy of the liver treatment for pernicious anaemia. After
this lecture we brought in some of these laudanum drinkers to
have a look at them and I found that they had no hydrochloric
acid in their stomachs. When I examined their blood they were
clearly cases of pernicious anaemia.

We began to give them hydrochloric acid in lemonade, a
shocking mixture to take, but it stopped the diarrhoea. Later,
when the Harvard treatment became known, they were made
to eat raw liver, which was not so bad. Some of them were so
far gone with subacute combined degeneration of the spinal
cord (a condition resulting from pernicious anaemia which had
not been treated and which had progressed to a dangerous
degree), that they were paralysed. As their anaemia improved
I had to teach them to walk again. This I did by tying a rope
across their backyards and marking out in whitewash, steps
on which they had to learn to put their feet. So they tottered
up and down their backyards holding on to the rope until
they were able to walk again, usually quite well.

Now and again perfectly beautiful cases turned up. One
Sunday a small man was brought by a group of little mountainy
types, his brothers, who carried him in, more or less invading
the surgery. I could see that he was very ill indeed. In fact he
seemed to be dying as he had a very acute fever, was pouring
sweat and was badly wasted. He had become ill about six or
more months before. He had been seen by his doctor, who
had sent him to the Royal Victoria Hospital in Belfast. There
they had diagnosed syphilis. His blood test was positive; there
was no doubt about it and that was that.

He was married, had a large family, and he was absolutely
certain that there was no way he could have contracted syphilis.
The people in the Royal did not believe him, neither did his

doctor and neither did his wife. She upped and left him, taking the children with her and returning to her parents. He sought refuge with his family which included a number of tough little brothers, fighting men, who took his part. A family feud started. The affair caused so much trouble in the small country community that something had to be done and the parish priest suggested that he should be brought to me. I examined him, and apart from the fact that he was very ill, I could not make out what was wrong with him, although his condition seemed to be too acute for syphilis. I examined him in every way I could and still could not make a diagnosis. Just when I was beaten, I stripped him completely and again went over him very carefully. I spotted a small scar on the front of one leg, a tiny little brown thing. He said that that was where a rat had bitten him. At a threshing after the harvest the year before, he had passed a stack of oats and a rat had jumped out into his open shirt, ran down his trousers and had bitten him before he could kill it.

I took two scrapings from the scar, and stained one and had a look at it under the microscope. I saw an unusual spirochaete, quite unlike anything I had seen before, but it was not the spirochaete of syphilis. I told the assembly that he did not have syphilis, and they were very pleased.

The next morning I went to Belfast and showed the slides to Sir Thomas Houston in the laboratory of the Royal Victoria Hospital and he could not identify it either. He sent it to London where it was found to be a rare Japanese spirocheate, Morsus Muris, carried by rats and giving the same results as syphilis for blood tests. Anyway, I cured the poor man and peace was restored. In some things in medicine, I have been very lucky. Other people who knew very much more than me had relied too much on scientific tests, and missed the rat bite. When one is up against a problem and there is no simple direct explanation, the sensible thing to do is to seek for an 'added dimension'. No one had ever stripped the patient before. In the Royal and everywhere else he had always been examined with the trousers of his pyjamas still on. In any case he was too ill or too stupid to tell them about the rat. In defence he claimed that no one had ever asked him about it.

In 1929 we began systematic ante-natal care for our mothers

which was quite a new concept. Till then, when a practitioner was called to a midwifery case, (most of which seemed to take place at night and in people's homes) he never knew what abnormality he might meet. The doctor, tired after a busy day, might not be at his best, his judgement could be impaired and the assistance from the midwife useless since in those days few were properly trained or qualified. If he met a serious complication the result could be devastating; the baby or even the mother could die.

There were no ante-natal X-rays and no blood transfusions; caesarian section operations were highly dangerous because of the risk of sepsis or of pulmonary emboli (blood clots forming in the pelvis and passing along to the lungs). Patients went into shock, which was a serious worry, particularly with poor, underfed mothers of large families. We knew very little about shock or how to treat it. One could meet toxaemia of pregnancy due to kidney failure and which could, in an extreme form, show itself as the dreaded eclamptic fits.

Of course doctors had great skill in the handling of the physical process of delivery, but even with this skill a large proportion of women were so mutilated that they were condemned to a lifetime of ill-health and discomfort if they did not undergo repair operations which meant more risk. Most midwives were untrained, in fact the Act registering them and attempting to bring them under some kind of supervision only became law in 1911. Some had traditional skills and were wise women but some were 'shockers', real Sarah Gamps. Luckily child-birth is a natural process and most women survived it. But far too many babies died in child-birth and the number of women losing their lives was disgraceful.

To introduce a simple scheme of ante-natal care into our practice was quite difficult. It was hard to persuade young women to submit to examinations to monitor their progress or to determine whether there was any abnormality present. If a problem was found, they were sceptical of the value of trying to do something about it, such as inducing an earlier delivery. The young ladies' mothers usually regarded this as 'interfering' and not natural. But, once we had it going, the scheme was of such tremendous value that I became a fanatic in promoting it.

On one maternity case I learnt a lesson which could be said to have influenced my life. One night I received a call to a case to the Montiaghs. The people were very poor and lived in a little cottage on a bit of cut-out bog. To get to it, I had to wade through a flood from the Lough. When I arrived I found that the patient was having a severe haemorrhage because the placenta was blocking the birth-passage.

There were half-a-dozen young children herded into another small room and an old 'handywoman' was in attendance and she was as usual, useless. I had two options, I could send the husband back through the flood to ride on his bicycle the few miles to the police barracks to ring for the hospital ambulance. She could well be dead by the time she got there, but everyone would say that 'Dr Jim, the moment he saw her, sent her to hospital and did his best'. I would be in the clear and could not be blamed. On the other hand, I could 'do a version', turn the baby and stop the haemorrhage. This was a serious procedure, and with a poor half-fed woman, she could well die. So I said a prayer, did the version and saved her. If it had gone wrong, all the water in Lough Neagh would not have washed me clean and for the next generation I would be haunted by that poor man and his six motherless children every time I saw them on the road. No woman's life should be at the mercy of such circumstances. Situations such as this are preventable; it is usually the poor who are the victims. Nowadays in Ireland, this kind of thing happens very rarely. This event, combined with other similar experiences, explains why I have such strong feelings on the care of women and children at birth and explains again why later on, I proposed the Mother and Child Scheme in 1946, as Chief Medical Advisor in the Department of Local Government and Public Health.

It is very difficult to describe the relationship which my father and I had with the community we served. It was not anything unusual, indeed it was more or less the norm for the old type of general practitioners. Lurgan was a 'soldiers' town. Whether it was the Crimean, Afghan, Boer or other smaller war of the Empire, the Lurgan men were always there. In my time it used to happen in this way. A boy leaving primary school at fourteen had only one hope, to be taken on somewhere as a message boy. Before the advent of telephones, small boys had one vocation only and that was to 'run messages'. When he became sixteen years of age and it was necessary to stamp his card for insurance he was let go and someone else taken on. If he was a Catholic (as people in this position generally were) he had then only one alternative, to go to the Depot of the Royal Irish Rifles in Armagh, lie about his age and enlist.

In a few months he would return, completely changed after regular good food for the first time in his life, drill, company and sport. He would swagger up the street with the green cockade of the Rifles in his beret and money in his pocket. After seven years he would be discharged and then, finding no work, would re-enlist for a further period and would end up as a corporal or sergeant and become a reservist. The result was that we had a tremendous number of army people, either sons, brothers or otherwise, of soldiers. Although complete rebels and treated shamefully, the Lurgan Catholics had tremendous pride in the two battalions of the 'Rifles' which in those days had a large number of Lurgan men.

On the fourth of August 1914, as a small boy, I remember the Catholic and Protestant men of Lurgan, for the one and only time in their history, marching together. When war was declared and the reservists called up, the Orangemen went to the lodges in the afternoon and took out the banners and marched around the town singing and the Catholics, a very much larger number, not to be outdone, went to the Hibernian Hall and took out whatever couple of banners they possessed and marched around too. Then the two lots joined up in great good humour and friendship for the first and last time in over three hundred years, and went off to the railway station and to the war. Most of them never came back; and for those who did, many of them would have been better dead.

Of all the many problem areas in our practice, that which affected my father most was the care of the veterans of the First World War. In all the unwritten histories of tragic groups, the men who returned from this war must be among the saddest. It is now more or less forgotten. Men who had endured weeks of shelling, living under dreadful conditions of hardship in dug-outs in the trenches, 'cracked-up' and were never the same again. They were labelled as 'neurasthenics' or 'shell-shocked' and lived out miserable existences in a kind of twilight of hopelessness. To survive they and their families depended on pensions.

Some had developed tuberculosis and become invalids. They sat about spreading the disease in the small workers houses. Many of those who served in Egypt came home with bilharzia and later developed bladder cancers. There were many with suppurating bone infections from gun-shot wounds. The British had a system of care for these unfortunates, backed up by hospitals and dedicated staffs, but what can you do for such people, crippled mentally and physically, particularly during a recession? The British Legion did what it could in generous hand-outs, but for the Catholics it was really not of much assistance.

In those days, politicians did not have clinics and the trade unions were rather feeble and so my father, without wanting it, became the defender of the ex-servicemen. Both Protestant and Catholic came under his wing. He became expert in applying for pensions for them or in having pensions regraded and in securing different benefits. In addition he gave them great medical care and they adored him.

One time they came to him and asked him to become a member of the County Council. He said that he was not interested as he was not a politician, disliked politics and would not canvass or try for election. They said to leave it to them and organised the whole campaign and my father was returned at the top of the poll as an Independent. They told him afterwards that they did it for the hell of it and to show him what they thought of him.

Of course I became indoctrinated into this kind of thing and became expert in my own right. It became more difficult to achieve anything for these men as the memory of the war receded. I remember one of my 'cases' with pride. This concerned a poor character who had never gotten anything because he had never been wounded or blown up, and looked the picture of health. He had a very considerable war service and had earned all kinds of medals.

After lengthy probing, I found that when his unit on one occasion had been almost wiped out, he had been some way or other linked up with a New Zealand crowd who had been similarly obliterated. Because his uniform had been destroyed he had worn a New Zealand uniform and been given a NZ pay-book. This was a major discovery. I found that after the Maori Wars, one of Queen Victoria's daughters, Princess Christian, had established a fund to care for British soldiers wounded or distressed after those long forgotten encounters. Even better, I found that there was some money left in the Fund. By the time I had finished a handsome ex gratia award was made to this poor Lurgan man. It made him happy for the rest of his life, even though he soon disposed of it on women, drink and foolishness. (In Lurgan 'foolishness' was regarded as a serious defect.)

On one occasion, when my mother was middle-aged, she had a vague illness and was not improving. She was not satis-fied with the local medical resources nor did any of the Belfast 'specialists' please her. So to satisfy her, my father took her to London to see a Harley Street specialist. I was taken too as I had won some small prize or other and had to be rewarded. I accompanied them to Harley Street, was introduced with pride to the great man as a medical student son, and then dismissed.

When we returned to Lurgan, my mother was to rest and receive some medicine. On her first day at home, she was rest-ing peacefully in bed in the afternoon, reading the newspaper and with her new medicine on the bed-table beside her. She dozed off and when she awoke, her medicine was gone. Later when he had finished the surgery, my father came up to see her and confessed that he had taken her medicine and had given it to some poor woman who was worse than she was and that he would replace it. I don't think she ever forgave him for that. One time later when she raised the matter, as she did quite frequently, she said that it had 'taken all the good out of her illness'. I tell this story as a typical example of what doctors used to be like and what were their relations with their patients.

There had been a history of violence and faction fighting in our town for at least three hundred years. For the last few generations it had been controlled fairly well by the old RIC and extra police were always drafted in to protect the Catholics during what is now called 'the marching season'. They were not always successful: on one occasion my great grandfather had to shoot out on an Orange mob who tried to 'burn him out' and as someone was killed, had to undergo trial. Indeed my father, as a magistrate, was the last person to read the Riot Act in Lurgan, in July 1907.

Up to the establishment of the Stormont government and for years after, the political interest of the Catholics was fairly harmless. The successors of the old Irish Nationalist Party paraded on 15 August under the banner of the Ancient Order of Hibernians but they were an ageing group and their cause excited little interest. They were seen to be quite ineffectual as a constitutional party since the Stormont Unionist government more or less ignored them.

However with the recession, the unemployment, the B-Special constabulary and the general tendency of the government to harass the Catholics there was a growing resentment, which ended up in the odd hot-head drifting into the IRA movement.

The B-Specials were a bit hard to take. On a night maternity case driving out to the patient's home in the country and coming round a corner, you would see a red lamp swinging in the dark on the road and a call to 'Halt'. Behind the hedges on each side of the road you were 'covered' by loaded guns handled by characters whom you knew well to be quite irresponsible. Then you were interrogated, your car thoroughly searched and you were sent on your way. You might be in a hurry on a serious case and to be held up several times like this was a nonsense, particularly since many of these people were my patients. In spite of efforts to exert discipline, they were quite likely to stage incidents; to keep things on the boil; a young Catholic fellow coming home on a bicycle from seeing his girl, being stopped, might give 'cheek' and be beaten up. Then of course the next day he would join the IRA.

During the war it was particularly galling for Catholics whose sons were in the Rifles, fighting Hitler, to have these well-paid characters, their neighbours, stopping them at road-blocks, searching them and generally strenuously and patriotically defending the Home Front, meanwhile letting them know who was boss.

This situation, as might be expected, created difficulties. For example, I was rung up on a Sunday afternoon by some unknown person and told to come at once to 'The Bacan MacAlindens', a cottage at the end of a very long lane where a blind man lived alone. Also, I was told to bring plenty of dressings. When I reached the place I found someone shot and wounded because a training exercise of young fellows for the IRA had been in progress and an accident had occurred. As I came up the lane, I saw people scattering and then a young man, a stranger whom I did not recognise, came forward and gave me orders on what I was to do with the wounded man.

I ended up telling him to go to hell and I put the wounded man in the car, lifting him in myself because he would not help me, and took him to hospital. Once in hospital I stayed with the patient and kept the police off him till he had had his operation and was fit to reply to their questioning. Then I received a polite request to visit the police station and was shown the bullet and asked a lot of questions on my part in the affair. It was easy to answer the questions because the young men concerned were smart enough to keep far away from me so that I could not identify anyone. That is how I believe I came to have a police record.

On my part, I did not agree with what the IRA were doing, had never joined them, had never fired a shot, in contrast to my great grandfather. I was a man of peace, but one did not let the side down. This of course was more than forty years ago and marked the beginning of the alienation of the minority which ended up in the serious troubles starting in 1969. I may also say that my view was universal amongst 'our side'.

It seems appropriate at this point to describe in some detail, the political and social situation in Northern Ireland during the period in which I was in practice in Lurgan.

When our country was divided, we the Nationalists who found ourselves on the wrong side of the Border, were outraged. Apart from the cynical injustice of providing a confessional state to suit a minority in the whole country, we were faced with a regime which was not likely to show us any mercy.

There was a monolithic association of Anglo-Irish landlords, big business in the form of the Linen-Lords, the various Protestant Churches, the Stormont Government, the Unionist Party, the Orange Order, the Royal Ulster Constabulary, the B. Specials, the Press, all inter-related, interwoven and acting in concert to preserve by every means they could think of, the Protestant Ascendancy. How totalitarian can you become? In fact, as carefully constructed instruments of state, which were the State, the whole thing from our point of view was an evil work of art.

For example, we were denied legitimate, democratic, political rights, by consumnate 'gerry-mandering' and artistic political corruption. There was no appeal from this situation, even though we were British citizens, since the Imperial Parliament at Westminster did not 'by convention' debate the affairs of Northern Ireland.

Even the Judiciary were affected. Though they may have tried to be impartial, the laws they implemented, such as the Special Powers Act, in force for fifty or sixty years, were corrupt insofar as they were really directed against Nationalism and the Nationalists. There was discrimination in housing, in jobs, and in social and cultural matters. For example, in our town of Lurgan, in the eight large factories in the town, one Catholic only was employed as a clerk. No Catholic had employment on the permanent staffs as administrator, manager, finance officer, skilled maintenance worker, tradesman or in any capacity, save as a work-floor 'hand'. And of course they were paid starvation wages. Many poor Protestants suffered as well, because of the corrupt, rotten system which divided the two communities, in the interest of big business, Unionist politics and control by Britain. Suffice to say, we became second-class citizens in our own country.

Of course they over-played their hand and as the Nationalists became better educated they questioned the situation and after forty years they demanded Civil Rights and the One-Man One-Vote issue occurred. It was civil and peaceful but was met by savage repression by the police. This was followed by the usual Orange pogrom and hundreds of Catholic homes were burnt out, people fled as refugees and there was accompanying sectarian murder of Catholics. The British Government sent in troops to protect the Catholics and the rule of Stormont was terminated. This was in 1969, and since then there has been twenty years of IRA violence, murder, bombing, and internment, military and police violence and torture, hunger-strikes and the Orange ascendancy still being maintained. People have a horror of the violence of the IRA but they forget that the IRA were the direct result of the '*Divide et Impere*' policy of Great Britain and of corrupt Orange Rule in Britain's first and last colony. I make no apology for them as I abhor violence and have been anguished for nearly twenty years of my life over the consequences.

You see, the last part of Ireland to be planted was the North, it was the most Gaelic and fought to the end. Most of the Planters were Scots, who were the same blood as we were, since they were descendants of the people who had founded the Irish Kingdom of Dalriada in Scotland and had Christianised the Picts. Over the three centuries that they have been here they have become thoroughly mixed with the 'native' Irish. As well, the Church of Ireland maintained a high-powered proselytising Mission all over Ireland for one hundred and fifty years and this was far more successful than people imagine and a tremendous number of the 'converts' ended up in the North. Look at the number of Murphys in the telephone book in the North, at the number of Church of Ireland Clerics and the Unionist politicians with Gaelic names and even count the number of Gaelic names on tombstones in St Mark's church-yard in Armagh, the heartland of Protestantism and you will see that we, the Northern people, are all one breed or at least so mixed that there is no difference between us, genetically, or by blood or birth or what-have-you.

The other thing is that these people, on both sides of the 'house' are the decentest people God made. I know, my prac-tice was half and half and I brought them into the world, saw them in all sorts of trouble and helped them when they died. To my father, brother and sister, they were neighbours and patients to be helped and we were concerned with them as people and not with their politics. I knew the Northerners and respected them and loved them and it has been dreadful to see them kill one another, torture one another, bomb one another and deny one another simple justice.

To be fair to the British, when they woke up to what was going on they terminated Stormont, tried to set up an As-sembly, tried to organise Sunningdale and power-sharing and the Anglo-Irish Agreement and have tried hard to create peace and harmony in the Province of Northern Ireland. But they have not prevailed over the Orange determination to maintain supremacy. As well they have really made something of a mess of it as they move one step forward and then two steps back. Some of their viceroys have been very decent men indeed and then there appears a shocker and things go backwards. Incidents on the ground, when they go bloody-minded are no help. Anyway, I can't expect to see the end of it but at least, because of the decency of the ordinary man and woman in the North, peace and justice will come.

An aspect of practice in Lurgan was the practical skills which the old medical people possessed and exercised in those days. My father taught me dozens of tricks and little skills which had been handed down. They were a kind of wisdom and 'quickness of the hand' which are almost lost to-day. I became quite adept at pulling teeth, because during the poor times, really poor people could not afford a dentist. It was a free job because they had nothing. Indeed for older people with loose teeth I learnt from my father the knack of pulling them with my fingers. It was easy once you got the hang of it.

We worked a six-day week, no half-days, three surgeries a day, a tremendous amount of midwifery and night work and took the whole thing in our stride. To get to the cinema was a treat, but it was necessary to go to the neighbouring town where you were not quite so well known. Otherwise, whoever sat next to you would seize the opportunity to discuss his or her aunt's constipation while you were trying to concentrate on Betty Grable or some such star in a gripping drama. Once my sister, Sheelagh, joined us in 1930 the work-load became easier.

But life was really very pleasant. As soon as I earned some money I bought a small and old sailing boat for Lough Neagh, the 'Duck' and had a lot of fun with it. Several mornings a week during the season, I would make my way to Hugh MacAlinden's on the Lough shore, just before dawn, wading through the floods to get there. 'Hughie' was a fisherman who lived on a little bit of land on a point sticking out into the Lough. He had been a friend of mine since I was a boy and was a wonderful character. Then we would go out in his boat to an island to await the dawn flight of the ducks. I got an old and safe horse and rode out and had the odd hunt. It had to be old and safe as my friends would not trust me with anything else. Sometimes, on a Saturday afternoon I slipped away and went for a hunt with the beagles which were kept by local weavers and were a traditional sport around Lurgan. I preferred this to the ordinary harrier hunt on horseback. I saved more money and bought the first of some really lovely sports cars which were the joy of my life.

But the greatest pleasure was the Armagh Rambler's Club. Rambler's Clubs were an old and enjoyable feature of life in the North of Ireland. They had been in existence for more than one hundred years and were something like the Pickwick club. Charles Dickens made fun of them, but they were not just a joke and had produced some world famous field naturalists and archaeologists.

The club was run by a most unusual man called T.G. Patterson. He had started off in life as a grocer's curate, was pretty well a self-educated person who ended up a great scholar. He was elected a Member of the Royal Irish Academy and received an Honorary Degree as Master of Arts from Queen's University. He was founder of the County Armagh Museum, one of the best local museums in these islands. Apart from all this, he was a thoroughly decent man and was beloved by all who knew him and was exceedingly good company. I used to slip away from the practice and go on outings with Patterson and his lot.

Once I discovered a kitchen-midden, when there was a collapse of part of the face of a bluff at Castor's Bay on Lough Neagh. It was interesting because it was under an old house where John Wesley stayed and where he preached when he came to Lurgan. This excited great interest among the group, especially when I was able to identify bones of red deer and other interesting things among the debris.

My father and mother had a house at Greenore in County Louth and we spent our holidays there. Poking around, I found, underneath a small mound near the shore, a souterrain. I crawled into the tunnel but when I got in a fair bit it started to come down all around me and I got out very quickly. I closed it up and left it alone after that.

Somebody, somewhere in the North, started a musical body called the Council for the Encouragement of Music and the

Arts, shortened to CEMA and I was the local chairman. It never got off the ground in Lurgan because the Protestants insisted on playing 'God Save the King' at the end of the concerts and the Catholics would not have it. Most of the good musicians were Catholics and the Protestants were excellent choral singers and together they really added up. The pleasant thing was that they got on very well together and liked one another. But there was so much wrangling that what was a really worthwhile effort ended in failure.

Exactly the same thing happened over the Hunt. The North Armagh Harriers were quite a good little Hunt and my brother Donnell was Master for years. When he had Hunt Balls, which were necessary to make a bit of money, there were rows because one side demanded the 'National Anthem', which the other side called a 'Party Tune'. So Donnell, who was in the centre of all this unpleasantness wound up the whole affair.

For very many years, Lurgan had a very good town soccer team, called Glenavon. They did very well and were known. For a long time both Catholics and Protestants played together happily and indeed my uncle, Leo Donnelly, won at least half-a-dozen Irish international caps playing for them. With the coming of the Six County set-up, things changed and the Catholics got fed up with being abused as regards their politics and parentage and so on and gradually pulled out and went off and played Gaelic football. That was the end of the sporting partnership of the two sides in Glenavon.

So this was my life. Hard work in the practice, lots of interests and a lot of fun. Not making very much money but enough to get by.

Since the trip to Vienna, I had become interested in flying, and about this time 1931, I had a chance to do something about it. In Aldergrove, not too far from Lurgan, there was an RAF Territorial Unit, called the Ulster Bombing Squadron. I proposed myself as a pilot and was accepted provisionally. The planes on which we trained were old Vickers Virginias. You sat up in the nacelles of these great old machines, all dressed up in flying gear, sitting upon your parachute, with the huge engines roaring away, behind and above you. The flying speed was all of eighty miles an hour.

I was coming along quite well, despite my parents' strong disapproval, when I was interviewed by a visiting Air-Commodore, before being accepted for a commission as a pilot-officer. The interview seemed to be going all right until he asked me what I did in civil life. As soon as he heard that I was a doctor, he turned me down. He said that it took six months to make a pilot and five years to make a doctor and that in the event of war, I would have to be a doctor. I agreed to become medical officer to the Squadron on condition that I should be able to learn to fly. It did not work out. I was expected to sit in the sick bay while flying was going on, particularly on Sunday mornings. After a time, sitting bored in the sick bay, reading the Sunday papers, and getting no flying, I quit.

The following year, 1932, was the year of the Eucharistic Congress in Dublin. This was a tremendous event for the country. One million Irish people prayed together. It seemed to give us some sort of international recognition and there was a spontaneous excitement of religion, carnival, achievement, fun and a wonderful feeling of all being Irish together and of what a great people we were.

The Bishop of Dromore, who knew our family well, arrived one day with 'privilege' tickets for the whole event for my father, mother and myself. This meant top-hats and morning coats and ringside seats. In addition, I was asked to take care of the Archbishop of Madrid and to collect him and see that he was at his seat on time. This meant that I could drive all over the place, with the police waving me on when they saw the official sticker on my windscreen. It paid to be a good solid Catholic bourgeois from the North as regards little bits of privilege in those days.

This period of my life was pretty wonderful. For one thing, the development of the practice as a partnership rather than being merely my father's assistant was satisfying. Sheelagh, who was excellent in the practice, soon married John Woods, a doctor from nearby Armagh. Then, most important, was the bliss of being in love, of marrying, the fun of showing off my bride, of setting up house and of the start of the companionship and happy strife, which has now lasted for more than fifty years.

2

The First Surveys

THIS happy situation of living next door to my parents, working with my father, constantly gaining experience and learning all he had to teach me, and enjoying my new life with my wife, did not last.

One day, in 1937, coming home from an outing with the Armagh Rambler's Club, I suddenly became aware that I was concerning myself, as an amateur archaeologist, with people dead and gone hundreds of years ago, while all around me was a growing amount of misery, sickness and poverty. Should I not be more concerned with the living than with the folk who perhaps a couple of millenia before had created the kitchen midden at Castor's Bay on the Lough? It was not an extraordinary conversion, but rather a notion that could have affected anyone.

There were several reasons why such a thought should have entered my head. One was the deterioration in the ordinary welfare of the Lurgan community. The recession which had begun in the US in 1929 had affected us badly and as the years went on deepened, so we had very serious and growing unemployment and poverty. Under the British panel system of health care, which had just been applied to the North of Ireland, all insured workers were provided with free health care, but their wives and families were not. With prolonged unemployment, people ran out of benefit and ceased to be eligible for free treatment.

With the best will in the world, politicians and bureaucrats can be beautifully and administratively mad. When times are bad, it is not the workers who need free care but their wives and children. The worse things get, the more people need care.

The situation occupied me on and off for weeks; and then one Sunday at Mass, I saw in the bench in front of me a row of children and the penny dropped. I saw how ragged they were, how thin and with so little subcutaneous fat, their hair dry and poor, the backs of their legs covered with chilblains and their bare feet blue with cold. It was real hunger. But what could I do about it?

At that time, little was known about nutrition, particularly malnutrition. I set about collecting all the information I could find on the subject: how to diagnose it, how to measure and assess it, particularly in the community. I was helped by the Royal Society of Medicine in London of which I was a Fellow.

The Librarian was a very decent man and supplied me with references and a bibliography. I tried out different methods of assessment and estimation on my patients and after a bit, when I had learned something I wrote a paper on it called 'The Assessment of Nutrition'. The *Journal of the Ulster Medical Society* published it in July 1938.

While nobody knew very much about nutrition, much less how to think about it scientifically and how it might affect places like Lurgan, the League of Nations had established a nutrition section to study and research the subject only three or four years before. People had of course been studying it in India where Sir Robert MacCarrison had carried out such magnificent work that he could well be described as the father of nutrition. MacCarrison came from Lisburn and was some sort of family connection of ours.

I had now built up a little knowledge of nutrition, but did not know what to do about it. One night I was doing a maternity case out in the Montiaghs again, in somewhat similar circumstances to the case I described before, in a little thatched cottage. There was a wait, so I sat down in front of a big turf fire and lit my pipe. I looked down and saw a heap of American magazines, which the brother of the man of the house, a New York policeman, had sent him. On top of the heap was a *Readers' Digest* and I opened it at an article which said 'Do it now'. This, in true *Reader's Digest* style, made the point that everyone had an ambition to do something or other which they kept putting off, either till they had saved enough or till the children were reared or whatever. The thing was to 'Do it now!'.

The next day, I 'did it now', by going off to Belgium, which was the one other place in Europe where there was a sizeable linen industry, to have a look at the Belgian linen weavers. My wife and parents thought I was crazy since it was November, but Gemma came with me and it ended up a pleasant holiday. Through Jack Heaney, a cousin of mine, who was a flax-buyer for some of the North of Ireland linen mills, I got to see the inside of quite a number of Belgian factories and to see the weavers at work. I visited them in their homes, their cafés, went into the local hospitals and discussed the patterns of disease with doctors and secured an overall picture. I was amazed to see the contrast between the well-fed, contented, well-housed, well-cared-for Belgians compared with my poor, half-starved people in Lurgan. The Lurgan weavers wove the finest linen in the world and the Belgians rougher, coarser products but the difference between the two groups of workers was a revelation.

When I returned home, I wrote to Sir John Boyd Orr of the Imperial Nutrition Institute in Aberdeen. This was an animal nutrition research centre for the UK and indeed the Empire, but had lately turned its attention to human nutrition. Sir John had commenced a National Nutrition Survey of the UK, possibly inspired by the fear of an impending World War II. I asked him if I might come to see his work and enclosed a copy of my paper. By return of post I received an invitation to come to Aberdeen. I received a wonderful welcome there, delightful hospitality and was shown everything, being driven around Scotland to see the teams at work. More important than anything I was encouraged to go ahead with some ideas I had.

So when I came back to Lurgan, I began a survey of male linen weavers. I carried out a clinical assessment of the nutritional state of the group and related this to a study of their economic and social backgrounds. Luck was with me a bit further, since Queen's had just appointed their first lecturer in statistics. This was Harold Booker of the London School of Economics. He was delighted to have someone seek his help with a project.

Then in Aberdeen, I met Hugh Magee who came from near Newry. He had just been appointed Nutritional Adviser to the Ministry of Health in London and was anxious to get some studies going. Hugh helped me by borrowing pieces of apparatus from different institutions, county boroughs and so on in England, things I could not make or buy myself.

The survey worked out very well. I brought in 202 linen weavers, typical of those working and not working and examined them by a very strict set of criteria. I found that by any reasonable standard, 54 per cent were suffering from malnutrition and showed definite signs of this clinical state. I found that the malnourished had lower incomes and larger families and that their children were more likely to be undernourished than those weavers with a better nutritional state. I wrote up the survey and sent it off to the *British Medical Journal* which promptly published it in February 1939. Without knowing what I was doing, I had carried out one of the first studies of malnutrition in a sizeable industrial community. Around the same time two poverty surveys were carried out in Belfast, one by a Presbyterian Church group and the other by a Methodist group. Both revealed incredible levels of poverty.

Great things were happening in the world and I wanted to have a share of the action. There was lots of excitement in Ireland too. Father Hayes of Tipperary, the founder of Muintir na Tire (The People of the Land), a rural self-help organisation in the Free State, had asked me to speak on nutrition to his meetings, which I did and I became very friendly with him. Father Hayes was a curate in Tipperary and without any help from his superiors had started this movement which was spreading fast throughout the country. I was very fond of Father Hayes and appreciated his great qualities. This was before the war, when we were all looking for something because of the awful social conditions that had come about mainly through the depression. We were all politically naive and indeed Father Hayes used to sit at his desk under a great signed photograph of Mussolini, without the slightest idea of what a scoundrel he was. Father Hayes had been on some kind of official visit to Italy and had met Mussolini who had captivated this simple little priest. I became interested in Stefan Radich, the Croatian rural social philosopher and read all his works.

I next carried out a study on married women with families, who worked in the linen industry, on somewhat similar lines to the first. My idea was to do three studies, of men, of women and of children. I brought in a group of two hundred mothers of families and found the same kind of thing as I found amongst the men. The women showed a greater range of signs and symptoms of malnutrition. The numbers of conditions such as anaemia and hydraemia were striking. The second survey was a better job than the first since I had gained in experience. In both surveys I related the clinical conditions of the men and women to the family income, how it was spent, the number of children and so on.

These two surveys were carried out late at night, when I had finished the evening surgery and the late round of calls, usually after 11 pm. It became a joke in the town, to see husbands walking up and down outside the house like strike pickets, waiting to escort their wives home when I had finished 'surveying' them.

As Harold Booker had returned to England and there was no other statistician in the North of Ireland, I sought the advice of Roy Geary of the Central Statistics Office in Dublin. A statistician was essential, not only to ensure that the material was properly handled from the statistical point of view and possibly to help with the design of the experiment, but, most important, to have the data machine processed.

The machine analysis of statistical material by automatic card sorting machines such as the Hollerith or the Powers-Samas had not long begun, but I knew something about it, so my surveys were carried out with this in mind. Although a very much over-worked and unusual civil servant and having to look over his shoulder all the time because of the unauthorised use of the machinery and of clerical time, Roy agreed to transfer my material to punch cards and to machine it. He also agreed to carry out the correlations and statistical analyses that were required. He made one proviso, that I should publish any results through the Statistical and Social Inquiry Society of Ireland, a venerable institution going back to the eighteenth century. I should add that without the consent, approval and indeed connivance of that delightful old man Stanley Lyon, the Director of the Central Statistics Office, Roy could never have accepted my work.

The study on the women, entitled 'Poverty as the cause of ill-health', was published in May 1939. Queen's University gave me a Masters degree in science for it.

The surveys were not done for fun or curiosity. The trade union people got to hear of them and the late Jack Beattie, the Labour MP, and at that time the sole opposition member attending the Stormont parliament, raised the matter. I had a most encouraging letter from the late Bob Getgood, District Organiser of the Transport and General Workers Union in Belfast which is reproduced among the illustrations in this book and of which, over forty years later, I remain proud.

About this time, I found a few cases of polycythaemia[1] and wished to see what effect vitamin C would have on the over-supply of red blood cells, which is characteristic of this disease. There was a rationale for this as vitamin C is a reduction/oxidation factor in the body and it might have an influence in the uptake of oxygen by the red-blood cells. It did not alter the blood-count very much but it did have an effect on the clinical picture. People who were very ill, confined to bed, felt immensely better, got up and indeed some ended up riding bicycles again. I never could understand why this happened but these people, who with the over-supply of blood were a dark red colour in complexion became much better in colour and felt lighter in their movements. I published a paper on this in the *British Medical Journal* in December 1940.

Then several pleasant things happened. Professor J.M. O'Connor, the Secretary of the Medical Research Council in Dublin, who was also Dean of Medicine in University College Dublin, asked me to call to see him. He asked who financed me and I said that I financed myself and then 'out of the blue' he said that the MRC had £200 to spare and they would give me this as a grant to buy apparatus. For me, such a gesture was marvellous. It was the first little bit of recognition I had received and with the money I bought a centrifuge.

In the same year, 1940, I had an invitation from the BBC to give a series of lectures on nutrition on the Belfast radio. However I turned these into something of more interest. The Lurgan working women were great people and from their number I was able to choose some really clever and witty

1. Polycythaemia is a blood disease of unknown origin, where the number of red blood cells increases, the blood becomes thick and patients darken in colour, become torpid, weak and incapacitated.

talkers. After I had finished my talk we would discuss a menu for a family for a week with a home economics lady. The talks were based on the assumption that you had £1 a week to spend on food and a husband and three children to feed — the question was how would you spend it to the best nutritional advantage? I had already examined the economies of the families of two hundred women in Lurgan and so I knew what I was talking about. The approach excited so much interest that we had hundreds of requests for our diet sheets from the north of Scotland right down to Cornwall. The BBC authorities were very pleased with the whole thing as it was quite new at the time.

The talks were hilariously down to earth, because the Lurgan working women did not let us preach nonsense. They knew what buying food, cooking it and feeding a family really meant. My part as the doctor and nutrition expert was anonymous, but in Lurgan everyone knew who it was and in the back streets people who had them brought out their radios and placed them on the window-sills of the houses so that all the neighbours could hear the local ladies broadcasting under the guidance of 'Dr Jim'. On the other hand, the Belfast medical establishment took a poor view of this enterprise. They submitted a panel of experts whom they felt should be used for any broadcasts concerning health. The thought of a Lurgan rebel getting his nose into the BBC was too much for them. However they were solemnly given auditions and voice tests by the BBC and that finished it.

We had a second series and then the BBC moved the whole thing to London where I believe it was the start for the 'Kitchen-Front', a war-time programme which was a great success.

In 1941, I was elected a Fellow of the Royal College of Physicians, unusual for a general practitioner. I was also elected a Member of the Royal Irish Academy and Chairman of the Mid-Ulster Division of the British Medical Association and a member of the North of Ireland Branch Council.

It was a time of endeavour, excitement, happenings and good luck. In terms of professional development, the concern with contemporary health problems and their relationship to social conditions was of importance, as was the beginning of the socio-medical surveys.

In 1941, Professor O'Connor of the Dublin Medical Research Council sent for me again and this time offered me £250. He suggested that I should employ a technical assistant with the money. Alan O'Meara, who was Professor of Pathology in Trinity College, recommended to me a young man called Eric Murdock, a Dubliner, who had just secured his BSc. I interviewed him on the steps of the Graduates Memorial Building in TCD and he came north and began work the next day. A short time before I had engaged John Rogan as an assistant in the practice, so I now had a team. I rented two rooms over a butcher's shop across the street as a laboratory and we were in business.

That year I had spotted some cases which I diagnosed as pellagra, a disease due to nicotinic acid deficiency, and had collected sixteen specimens. People with this condition had eczematous changes on their hands and faces, and other areas exposed to the sun. They were anxious, nervous, listless and in really bad cases became so ill that they died. The condition had not been reported in Ireland before, so I wrote up the cases and published them in the *British Medical Journal* in January 1942.

That really started something. The day after the article appeared, a Saturday, I found two telegrams on the hall table. One was from Sir Jack Drummond of the Ministry of Food in London and the other from Hugh Magee of the Ministry of Health. Both said the same thing, that Professor Sydenstricker of the Rockefeller Foundation was in London and would like to come to Lurgan to see my cases.

I took the two telegrams in to my father next door and found him reading the newspaper before his lunch. When he had read them, he looked over his spectacles at me and said 'you are caught now, my boy'. This is how the great young medical scientist was regarded by his own father! It was, of course, the typical pawky Lurgan and indeed North of Ireland way of looking at things.

Sydenstricker duly arrived, bringing his slit-lamp with him and for two days examined my cases very carefully. Sydenstricker was ordinarily a very silent man, and for those two days he said nothing. Finally, I could not stand it any longer and burst out, 'They are pellagra, aren't they?' Whereupon Sydenstricker, the greatest authority in the world on the disease, finally spoke. 'They just could not be anything else but pellagra' he said. You could have heard my sigh of relief all the way out to the Montiaghs.

At that time I did not realise that during the Serbian Campaign in the First World War there had been a very severe outbreak of pellagra and a great number of people had died. Whitehall were worried about it and had asked the Rockefeller Foundation to send them Sydenstricker. During his first week in London my paper had appeared, so they sent him over to confirm whether this was the beginning of a major out-break. However it was a small localised thing and with treatment, which had not been available in the Serbian situation, I soon cleared it up.

Sydenstricker became a good friend of ours and in consequence of whatever he said about his trip, other Rockefeller people came later to see what I was doing. Sydenstricker's visit had been reported to the Northern government by Whitehall and Dr McCloy, the Chief Medical Officer of the Belfast Ministry of Health, came down to Lurgan to see him. He said that the people in Queen's and the Royal Victoria Hospital staff had prepared a programme for him. I said that Professor Sydenstricker's programme had already been arranged and he asked 'who had done this, was it Whitehall?' and I said 'no, I did; after all he had come to see me'. Sydenstricker was very amused at all this and entered into the spirit of the thing. When they asked him to dinner at the Reform Club in Belfast, he would not go until I received an invitation as well. So I found myself dining with all my former teachers, the whole Medical Faculty of Queen's, in a place I had never been or was ever likely to visit. Politics, bigotry, intolerance and being on the wrong side of the fence interfered in everything in those days in the North of Ireland. On the other hand, I found that these hard, stern-faced people were really friendly human beings and that when they had lowered a few drinks could become as lively as crickets.

With Eric Murdock and John Rogan, I began a series of studies on ascorbic acid. First, to confirm whether it (vitamin C) was related to complement[2] and thus played a part in the body's resistance to infection. This was in all the text-books but there did not seem to be any scientific evidence for it. It seemed to have crept in and to have been copied from one text-book to another. We found that ascorbic acid, whether or not it played a part in resistance to infection, did not do it because of its relationship to or influence on complement. We published this finding in the *Irish Journal of Medical Science* in March 1943.

Next we studied the excretion of ascorbic acid at different levels of the substance in the blood, from saturation down to scurvy levels. We dieted ourselves for weeks and took blood samples at the different levels, on different groups of days, every three hours. We found to our surprise that we were still excreting ascorbic acid even when we got to the scurvy level. That was interesting because man and the guinea pig are the only mammals which were believed to have lost the ability to synthesise vitamin C in the body and so are dependent on external supplies of fruit and vegetables. Yet here were we, with the substance gone from our blood streams, still excreting it. We published this result in the *Irish Journal of Medical Science*.

At Mass one Sunday, when I should have been thinking of higher things, I got an idea for a test for ascorbic acid in whole blood, which it had not been possible to estimate before this. We published this test in the *Biochemical Journal* in March 1943. This list of things is history now, forgotten and mouldy but it was fascinating at the time.

Although we were very lucky, it was not roses all the way. We started many things that we could not finish. We might come to a dead-end and have to take another line, which again might not work out. We learnt from these mistakes, but nothing could eliminate the helplessness of the old-time doctor in the face of many problems. Too often the bacteria beat all their work. For me it was an increasing disillusionment that pushed

2.   Complement is the name given to a group of proteins present in normal blood serum. They play a complicated part in the body's immune defences. Complement dissolves or haemolyses sensitised blood cells, has bactericidal, bacteriolytic and other important functions.

me into public health. What we published were the things that we had worked through and there was much of our research which never saw the light of day.

Eric got a PhD working in the team, and more or less grew up in Lurgan, changing from a shy young student to a positive, determined character who went on to have a very successful career as a chemist with Unilever. John Rogan was a first-class physician and an excellent colleague.

What I have just described were more or less the routine things, but there were exciting moments. I had been testing people who were cyanosed (bluish hands and faces) from heart and chest conditions, I gave them ascorbic acid and by using various alkalis was able to raise the level of the substance in the blood considerably. It improved their colour and symptoms in quite a remarkable way and I was trying to find out how it worked.

One day, in the neighbouring town of Banbridge, when coming out of a house where I had been seeing a patient, I noticed on the other side of the street a 'blue man'. I said to the daughter of the house who was seeing me out, 'That's an interesting fellow, I'm working on this kind of thing at the moment and if it comes out it might help people like him some day'. She replied that she knew him, that he had been like that all his life, that he had been investigated all over the place in different hospitals and that there was no cure for him. Anyway, we left it at that.

About ten days later, he came to my surgery in Lurgan one wet winter's night. The place was full of patients waiting, so I took him across the road to Eric who was working in the laboratory and told him to give him a cup of tea and keep him in chat till I could find the time to get over to see him. I rang his doctor in Banbridge and got his agreement to my treating him. Later I went over and took a big blood sample, but he unfortunately 'passed out'. We had quite a job to get him well enough to face the journey back to Banbridge. I gave him some ascorbic acid and told him how to take it. As I had a couple of patients to see in Banbridge the next week I said I would call to see how he was getting on and that I would need another blood specimen. He said that he did not want me to come to his house, and when I asked why he answered in a

shamefaced way, 'Well, you know what you are' meaning
that I was a Catholic. Eric, a Dublin Protestant, exploded
when he heard this. Anyway, we arranged to meet at the 'tank
barrier' outside Banbridge the following Sunday morning
while his people were at the Presbyterian Meeting House. Eric
and I duly turned up and 'your man' arrived in a little Austin
Seven car.

He got out and came over to us and low and behold, he was
nice and pink and the blue colour had gone. He said 'what do
you think of me?' 'If you weren't such a bigoted bastard', I
answered, 'I could kiss you'. Then he wanted to know would
he stay pink and various other questions. Just as he was leaving
he came back and asked could other people take those tablets
for as he said 'my brother is blue too'.

Since the whole business was so interesting, I rang Professor
O'Connor and he suggested that I should bring the two men
down to Dublin and accompanied by Eric Murdock we arrived
at Professor O'Connor's laboratory in UCD. He had gathered
together there some of the bright young medical stars of
Dublin. I remember D.K. O'Donovan and Oliver Fitzgerald.
What I had found were two cases of familial ideopathic methae-
moglobinaemia. This was a rare blood disease and I had found
the first cases in Great Britain or Ireland and the third recorded
in medical literature. So far as we knew, these were the first
to be cured, or at least to have their colour changed.

It was arranged that I should treat the second lad under the
eyes of Douglas Harrison, the Professor of Biochemistry and
Henry Barcroft, the Professor of Physiology of Queen's University. Henry Barcroft had an artist match the colour of the
skin every day as he changed from blue to normal pink. We in
Lurgan treated the patient and did our tests and so did the
professors and everything went well. Shortly after I published
a paper on the cases in the *British Medical Journal* in June
1943. It was picked up by the international newsagencies and
came back to the Irish papers via the wire services.

For a few days I was famous. Letters came from 'blue'
people everywhere, and some were pathetic. There was the
'blue lady' in St Stephen's Green in Dublin. This was an elderly
silver-haired lady who used to sit in St Stephen's Green resting
in the sun. I could not do anything for her. Many years before

a doctor in Dundalk used to treat his epileptic patients with silver nitrate tablets. Why, I never found out. Silver nitrate is stored in the body, where it accumulates. When there is enough, the parts of the body exposed to the sun undergo a chemical change in the skin, exactly like a photographic plate and so these people become a slate-grey. The change is irreversible. I came across other cases of this extraordinary treatment by this unusual Dundalk doctor, who is long since dead as are all his patients.

Douglas Harrison later put one of his assistants, Quentin Gibson, a very bright young man, to work on methaemo-globinaemia and he pushed along knowledge of the condition quite a bit and gradually interest grew and more and more work was done on it. Harrison and Barcroft wrote papers and more cases came to light and knowledge increased. Shortly after this, and up to a point parallel with our work, it became possible to employ new techniques and by the use of x-ray diffraction methods Max Perutz and John Kendrew, working with haemo-globin and myoglobin respectively, worked out the molecular structure of haemoglobin and myoglobin. Between 1950 and 1960 they were able to prepare three-dimensional models in which every atom was in place and the structure was a helix. In 1962 they shared the Nobel prize for their marvellous work. This triumph of Perutz's required the placing of 12,000 atoms in the helix and this was one of the first proteins whose mole-cular structure was completely worked out.

Anyone working in science, no matter how primitive or elevated, must preserve a proper sense of humility. Sometime later it was found that a decent country-woman living in the middle of the County Tyrone had a family with some 'blue' children. She found that when she fed her 'blue' children with cabbage, they became nice and pink. When she stopped, they became 'blue' again. So they got plenty of cabbage to eat. But she never won a Nobel prize.

Our home as I have said was in a row of houses built by my great-grandfather and the last house, owned by my aunts, had been requisitioned by the Army to become the residence and the Headquarters mess of the General Officer Commanding the British Army in Northern Ireland. Later when the American 5th Army came to Europe, they took over the house in turn and General Collins, the Commanding Officer of the 5th US Army, lived there and had his HQ staff Officers Mess.

The Senior Chaplains were billeted on my mother and father and the thing spilled over to our house, again 'next door'. We ended up with all kinds of senior officers coming in to put our children to bed and the place was swimming with candy bars and orange juice and what have you. There was a nightly poker game in my father's house and gradually we came to know all these very fine people. The whole thing was a most unusual experience for people like us, who had never had this kind of treatment before.

My father had not been too well, and needed a rest as his heart was not the best and retreated to the house we had at the sea in the County Louth. There he had another circle of friends and played bridge. One of his close friends was Cardinal Mac-Crory, whom he had known for many years and who had a house nearby. One afternoon in 1942, the Cardinal arrived in distress. In August some six young men had been condemned to death for the shooting of a policeman. The policeman was a decent soul, the boys were young and the whole thing was sad. It excited great public interest in the North and indeed in England and all kinds of people who had no interest in politics became concerned. The Cardinal had had several appeals from people to do something to save these youngsters, who were about to be hanged. He wanted to talk it over with my father as he did not know what to do. Between them they cooked up the idea that there should be an appeal to the American Forces for clemency for the condemned. They dithered about it for a while until my father said 'Jim knows the American General'. I was sent for and deputed to ask for an interview with General Collins and to ask him to allow any of his officers who so wished, to sign a petition for clemency.

Anyway, I went home to Lurgan and saw the General in Brownlow House, the World Headquarters of the Orange Order, the former home of Lord Lurgan, where I had danced many a night at Rugby Club dances. Before seeing him, I had to tell him what I wanted to see him about and when I got there he sat at a table with a row of senior officers and also an RUC officer, which worried me.

I presented my case, but he was reluctant to commit any

of his officers to any kind of interference. He stated that they were there and enjoying hospitality from the North of Ireland government and then launched into a speech on the iniquities of the Nazis and so on. I listened and it was obvious that he was not going to allow anything, but something he said upset me. Now at that time, I was a really impudent 'pup' and was not overawed by any American general. So I told him that the Orangemen whose headquarters he was sitting in, were, from our point of view, quite as bad as the Nazis. That there was no use going to Germany or whatever to fight an enemy when he had it on his door-step and so on. He got very mad; the only thing that saved me was the fact that his officers were quietly splitting their sides at my 'cheeking' their general. Some of them might have been of Irish origin. He turned to the RUC officer and asked him had he anything to say to this and he said 'no', but I am sure that it went down on my record. He then threw me out politely and went on to other business with his officers. In the end the young men weren't hanged.

While the 'blue' men business was good, clean, amusing, if primitive, scientific fun, the next job we did I regard as being of far more significance. I decided to carry out an Infant Mortality Survey of Belfast. This was to replace the study originally intended on the Lurgan children. I had 'done' the parents and there did not seem much point in following this with a children's survey, since I should simply find the same thing, that they were malnourished. In any event the war had changed the picture.

The Second World War provided an abundance of work, and people earned plenty of money. It was interesting to see that the Lurgan people had been so inured to poverty and hardship that even the worst war-time conditions were regarded as luxury. People had work and money in their pockets and were much better paid. The poor characters whom I had attended over the hungry years and who had had no money to pay me came along and not only paid what they thought they owed but said 'thank you' when they got into work and started to earn.

Even to-day infant mortality is a problem in Belfast. Forty years ago it was dreadful. Writing in 1943, I pointed out that for years more than one child in every eight had died during the first year of life. Very little was known about the causes, and with all the political, social and health problems of the day, little was being done about it. We did not advertise our project. If we had, the establishment would have tried to find some way or other to stop us. We just went ahead and did it.

One of the good things about the North of Ireland is the number of really decent folk with social consciences who will go to endless trouble to help with something in which they believe. The Registrar General of the North of Ireland, W.A. Carson, was one of these people and he was delighted to see his records put to positive use. He quietly dug out for us the names and addresses of all the Belfast babies who had died between June 1941 and June 1942. This group numbered five hundred and fifty-four. Then we took a control group, which included every fifth child born during the period, and which had survived. This group enabled us to compare those who had lived with those who died.

We then called at each house and interviewed the mother and discussed the life of the child, the illness history, particularly the last episode, the care the child had received, the feeding it had been given and noted the domestic efficiency or cleanliness of the house, the district, the occupation of the parents and a lot else besides. It was extraordinary how clear people were about the circumstances relating to each death. Mothers remember every detail.

When it is appreciated that this study was done during the war and with war-time conditions of transport and all the other inconveniences, it can be seen that it was quite a task. We visited the houses of all those children. While I went to the houses myself in the beginning to organise the protocol, the vast bulk of the visiting was done by Eric Murdock on his bicycle. As often as not, he rode the twenty miles to Belfast, went round the houses then back twenty miles to Lurgan. Eric's tact, patience and hard work in securing these interviews was remarkable.

Roy Geary's staff in the Central Statistics Office in Dublin carried out the punching of the cards, sorted them and prepared the tables. Roy did a superb job in analysing the material and preparing mathematical correlations between the various factors that we had investigated. The field work was finished in February 1943 and we published the results in a paper in the *Journal of the Statistical and Social Inquiry Society* in

May 1943. We published two other papers, one in the *Ulster Medical Journal*, dealing with what we thought should be done about the problem. The other was in the *British Medical Journal* and considered infant feeding in relation to mortality and showed that the failure to breast feed infants was significantly related to the high death rate.

The main findings of the survey were that the babies who died were almost a pre-selected group. The babies who lived, thrived in an exuberant way, were rarely ill and were more often well breast-fed than those who died. The babies who died had a lower birth weight. The parents of these babies mainly lived in the poorer areas and had smaller incomes than the rest. General practitioner medical care was usually adequate but no trained nursing was available to deal with the sick children. The ordinary public health nursing service of those days was ineffective in dealing with really sick infants. The babies who died lived in smaller and more over-crowded houses. There was a lack of coordination in the health services. The main causes of death were respiratory infections, gastro-intestinal conditions, premature births (low birth weights) and a group of miscellaneous disorders. Even in those days, I was convinced that seventy per cent of those five hundred and fifty-four babies could have been saved.

We also had a tremendous problem of tuberculosis in the practice. For example, there were young adults developing miliary or 'galloping consumption' and who were dead within a few months of their first being seen. In their case the tubercle bacilli found their way into the blood stream and were disseminated all over the body. A mother would bring in a young teenager and say that she had not been well lately. You would notice a high flush on her cheek-bones, even a slight bluish tinge and a shortness of breath. Her eyes would seem brilliant and even an ordinary child would appear to have an odd beauty. The temperature would be raised and when you examined the lungs you would hear the little whispering rales which could only mean one thing, that she would be dead in a month or so.

There were pensioners from the First World War, who suffered from tuberculosis, sitting around and infecting adolescents and in particular, babies, and causing amongst them a lot of TB meningitis. Children suffering from tuberculous peritonitis, lay in bed with great white swollen bellies, and the only treatment was to wrap them in flannel soaked in cod-liver oil and iodoform. The stink of this mixture in the small workers' houses was dreadful. There was little or no control of milk hygiene, and cows infected with TB, particularly if they had udder abcesses, distributed the disease far and wide. The result was a very large number of cases of bone and joint TB. There was a range of TB hips, spines, knees and infected glands in the neck, otherwise known as scrofula or the 'King's Evil', all to be seen. Conditions unknown now, such as TB dactylitis, where a child's fingers swelled up and a hand would look like a bunch of evil, deadly-white parsnips were seen. All over the place you could spot hunch-backs and old TB hips where the bone had shortened and caused deformity and such people were on a crutch and were known as 'crutchies'. And of course there were large numbers of people with chronic suppurating abcesses and sinuses from bone disease.

Cases were treated with fresh air and anything which might build up the appetite and health of the sick person. Some surgical procedures were of value in the odd bone case. Occasionally it was possible to isolate them in our little local sanatorium at Armagh, but it was feared as a 'death house' from which few ever emerged alive. I tried gold injections, calcium and all kinds of things. The older doctors believed in tuberculin injections, by which they tried to raise the patient's resistance. There was a great mystique about this treatment, but I found it to be useless.

Back in 1927, a recently established radiologist in Belfast called Richard MacCullough, had begun to x-ray chests for TB and outside his specialty but using x-rays to control what he was doing, carried out pneumothorax treatment for lung tuberculosis. He inserted a cushion of air between the chest wall and the affected lung so that it collapsed and was rested and enabled to heal. He gave us a lecture on his techniques. Partly influenced by the delightful, warm personality of Dicky MacCullough, whom I got to know, and because this was a hope in the bleak outlook for tuberculosis patients, the following year when I qualified I had decided to try this for myself.

There was an old First World War x-ray set in Lurgan Hospital. It was an exciting machine and spat out huge blue electric sparks all over the place. Dr Tom Pedlow, a decent man who 'did' the x-rays, let me move it away from the wall of the room where it was housed, so that I could get sufficient penetration and we began to do chest x-rays for TB.

Originally it was really to study the matter and to see how one could use it for diagnosis. At first I did not know or appreciate very much what I was seeing, but gradually I learnt and began to carry out pneumothorax or lung collapse myself. In those days things were far more easy and flexible than they are now. To-day, the idea of a young, newly qualified practitioner going into a hospital x-ray department and starting to move things around, just would not be tolerated.

Fifty years ago, one of the problems of tuberculosis was the lack of knowledge on how the disease spread and what were its characteristics as an epidemic. In order to get a picture of the disease as it affected the community of Lurgan, I went through all the death certificates of people who died during the previous twenty-five years and picked out those who had died from tuberculosis of one form or another. I noted when and where the deaths had taken place and plotted them out on Ordnance Survey maps.

What I found was that slow epidemics had occurred, particularly, as could be seen, in working-class houses and working-class streets. These would persist in one or more adjacent houses or streets and after a few years burn out and start up again in another district. It showed a geographical 'clustering' of the disease over a period and I called it 'slow-motion contagion'. It was a rough simple kind of study but to me it was very illuminating. From my knowledge of the place and its people it was obviously accurate. It also offered information on the people at risk and who needed to be protected, if at that time it were possible.

During the spring of 1943, it was apparent that the practice was growing bigger all the time and my father was growing older. John Rogan our medical assistant was very good but it was obvious that soon we would not be able to cope. I would work hard all day and late at night go across to the laboratory and stay there till about three in the morning, and perhaps as soon as I had gone to bed, have to go out to a maternity case. There was also the difficulty of war-time conditions, driving in the 'black-out' and so on. We worked Saturdays and Sundays as well. I was neglecting the family who were being sacrificed to my dedication to work. Since we 'lived over the shop' they did see me every day but for a few minutes only and at long intervals.

When I took holidays, we moved the show down to Dublin, where Percy Kilpatrick, the Registrar of the Royal College of Physicians gave us a room to work in and we would work all day, punctuated by visits to the bar of the old Wicklow Hotel for food and drink. We went to Dublin to have peace to write up the papers and to be near Roy Geary and the machines in the Central Statistics Office. We lived like this till we got the various jobs done.

After 1939, each year a group used to organise a Social Order Summer School in Clongowes, my old school. These gatherings were at that time a major event in the intellectual life of the country. They were great fun, you met everybody, argued day and night and learnt a great deal. Sandy MacGuckian, a Northern agricultural genius, and I used to go together. However after a few years, at an open session, I asked one of the principal speakers, the Bishop of Galway, Michael Browne, a formidable man 'what was the Church's view on the attitude of a Catholic in the North of Ireland to the government of Northern Ireland?' He answered that 'as the government of Northern Ireland was an effective, de facto, legitimate government, a Catholic had the duty to give it respect, obedience and loyalty'.

On the same day, I got into an argument with Dr O'Neill, the Bishop of Limerick, a former President of Maynooth. I pointed out that there were some twenty thousand priests and nuns in Ireland, all educated to a third level and I asked what had they done to improve the social situation of the country apart from teaching and some nursing. He said that a priest's job was to preach the Gospel and not to act as a social worker. While he was largely right, I did not think that the matter ended there and so the argument grew to be hot and heavy. However he held his ground. After these two incidents, I felt that the atmosphere was not right for me and I did not go back.

The National Health Insurance Authority of the Free State asked me to help with some research. The Chairman was

Dr Dignan, the Bishop of Clonfert and they had Rory Henderson as Secretary, a most enlightened pair. Rory O'Brolchain
was a kind of research assistant and he was both intelligent
and knowledgeable in social affairs. As well, they had an excellent battery of statistical machinery, which was just up my
street. I did some studies for them, analyses of their sickness
experience and investigations into some of their problems with
unusual disease patterns and other such things. I remember
one job in which I compared the sickness experience of Dundalk and Drogheda, two neighbouring and comparable towns.

I became a member of the Northern Ireland Branch Committee of the British Medical Association in 1941/2. As Chairman of the Mid-Ulster Division, I attended various committees
as an ex-officio member. At one of these meetings, the Chairman and Secretary of the whole Northern Ireland Association
told us that they had visited the Ministry of Health by invitation, met the Minister, and had agreed more or less on a new
plan for the Health Services. Here it was and would we please
approve of it. Although I was the most junior member there,
I felt outraged that they had done this without telling us and
got to my feet and said what I thought. I sat down thinking
that I had made a fool of myself and that as a Catholic I would
be regarded as following the usual line of stirring up trouble
and that I should have kept quiet. To my surprise I was followed by nearly everyone present and they said the same thing
and they ended up proposing a vote of 'no confidence' in the
office-holders. Whereupon, there was a new committee voted
in and I found myself on it and in turn was elected to represent
the North of Ireland on the Central Practitioners Committee
in London. I never attended a meeting, since I left for Dublin
soon after.

Great things were happening in the world, so I went off to
join the British Army. My application was referred to the
North of Ireland War Services Committee, Medical Section.
This was mainly staffed by the establishment and particularly
the people whom I had helped to vote off the British Medical
Association Council. So I was offered a commission as General
Duties Lieutenant. This wasn't good enough and MacCarrison
and Magee recommended me to the War Office as a Nutrition
Specialist and W.J. Wilson, my teacher, recommended me as a

Public Health Specialist as I had the DPH, but it came back to the same group and they did not approve. I went to join the Free French and they blocked that too and also I had a shot at UNNRA and the same thing happened. One never knew what was behind things in the North, possibly I might have had a police record for the odd inadvertent mix-up with the IRA, without knowing it. Then they graciously made me Chemical Warfare Officer for Lurgan, where I picked up the formula for DDT, which came in handy later.

I was not idle, since the Ministry of Food and the Ministry of Health in London frequently used me as a kind of unofficial advisor on nutritional matters in Northern Ireland. I remember one job was a kind of regular estimation of the level of vitamin B in the population. I would take blood samples either at random or from selected groups whom I thought might show a deficiency. Eric Murdock would take them on his bicycle to Stormont and they would go to Whitehall in the Home Office mail bag. They would be sent by motorbicycle courier to Sir Rudolph Peters' laboratory at Oxford. This Home Office mail bag was a great lark. I had a line on a wonderful stock of Old Comber whiskey, a distillery which had ceased to function but which had made the most wonderful malt. So as often as not, there were bottles of the aforesaid whiskey labelled as 'medical samples for analysis' for the poor benighted people in the Ministry of Health and the Rockefeller Advisers in Curzon Street. Now and again they would send for me and I would arrive loaded down with blood and other 'specimens'. I can still dimly remember a party in Curzon Street, which followed one of my arrivals, while the odd bombs were falling all around.

During the few years before 1944, things had begun to change in medicine and it affected us in Lurgan. One was the introduction of the first 'sulpha' drug, Prontosil (Bayer). This had a magical effect on the streptococcus and in puerperal sepsis. It was fascinating to see it cure women as if by a miracle, women who would otherwise have died. Another drug, M & B 693 was equally dramatic in saving lives in the pneumonias.

The local hospital had been reconstructed in 1936 and under my class-fellow Bill Basset provided a completely new standard of modern surgical service. The difference that Bill's energy and ability made was a revelation. One enormous advantage to our practice was that we were allowed to treat our obstetric patients in the private and semi-private maternity wards. The cost of the semi-private wards was so low (£2 per week) and the service so good, that with the coming of the war and the fact that the people now had money, every woman could afford the accommodation. With a good ante-natal service and this amenity, our maternity care was transformed, and I could feel that we were able to give our patients a really good service; the old nightmares and terrible dramas were ended. Bill Basset never received nearly enough recognition for the great job he did in Lurgan.

In the summer of 1944, the post of Chief Medical Adviser to the Department of Local Government and Public Health in Dublin was advertised and I applied. At the interview I was asked 'Had I any administrative experience?' and when I said that I had not, was more or less dismissed. But no appointment was made and the post was re-advertised. I decided that I had no chance of the job and was about to ignore it, when my father received a very mysterious letter from a former classmate, whom he had not met for nearly forty years. It said that he was aware that I was interested in the post and that he should encourage me to re-apply. So I applied again, had a better interview this time, when they encouraged me to talk and so I was appointed. At the same time an offer came of a post to look after a Jewish Refugee Camp in North Africa and the North of Ireland War Services Committee felt that this was suitable for me, so I had a choice of two jobs to go to. Sadly but perhaps wisely, I chose the Dublin post.

While I had been quite light-hearted at the idea of leaving Lurgan, when it came to the point things were different. After sixteen years of practice in the town where I had been born and in which I had grown up, I had become so involved with the people, so concerned and fond of them that to have undergone the usual prolonged leave-taking would have been unbearable, so I just vanished. One day I was at work in the practice, the next sitting at my desk in the Custom House in Dublin.

I learnt how easy it is to be 'done without'. After sixteen years during which I had participated in the lives of the people of the town and the country around, in births, deaths, happenings, crises of all kinds, things went on as before. It was as if I had never been there.

It was not so bad for the patients as my brother Donnell, a good doctor, who had been serving in the Irish Army, had just been released and could take my place. Also the situation had altered, the war-time care of children with allowances, food-supplements, the atmosphere of work and plenty of money had changed everything. Even with war-time conditions, the antibiotics and the excellent hospital and the special provision for maternity care had made the practice a much more pleasant occupation.

3

Early Days in the Custom House

C oming to Dublin was wonderful. For the first time I discovered my country. I suddenly felt a free citizen of a free country and began the process of getting the repression and bitterness of the North out of my system. Everybody had opinions and expressed them, and to me the atmosphere was heady. You could move anywhere at any time and not be held up and questioned by the B Specials. You were not the recipient of the odd quiet warning to watch what you said and so on.

I also had to learn and understand the interactions and tensions between political parties, personalities, trades unions, the churches, civil service, the Anglo-Irish and between institutional, professional and other factional interests. I had to realise that I was witnessing a national democracy in place of what I had hitherto experienced, the one-party, long-continuing repressive, fascist-type rule in the North.

The second thing I discovered was that I was now a member of an organisation, the Department of Local Government and Public Health, with rules and regulations, division of labour, with responsibility for staff, and that I was no longer a freelance. My freedom of action was likely to be restricted.

The third thing was that after sixteen years of practice in my own town and fairly well on top of the job, I was suddenly starting on a new career with major responsibility and without the support of family, friends, patients or my lifetime environment. It meant finding a new home in Dublin, which was likely to be difficult with war-time restrictions. The new job also represented a considerable drop in income. I had to face the possible resentment as an outsider appointed over the heads of senior people, already in the service and quite competent to fill the post and with reasonable expectations of succeeding to it. I was not identified in any way with any

party or political view, had no 'national record', had graduated
from a Northern university, had never worked in the Free
State, had never held any kind of official job before, knew
nothing about administration and did not speak Irish. My
whole history to date had been that of a loner, a freelance
and possibly a maverick.

Sitting alone in my room in the Custom House, the beautiful building inhabited by the Department of Local Government
and Public Health, I thought of all these things and became
so concerned that I seriously wondered whether to go home.
Thinking it over, however, there were things in favour of staying as opposed to the adventure of going off to North Africa
to look after the Jews. The job had a prestige title, though
without being all that powerful. Further, all the things I had
done in the years before had really fitted me for the post.

For example, there was the enormous problem of maternal
and infant mortality in the state. I had personally carried out
more than 5,000 deliveries, had organised an ante-natal service
in Lurgan and, even more important, had conducted one of
the first Infant Mortality Surveys anywhere, so I knew quite
a lot about the subject. On tuberculosis also, I had quite a lot
of experience, whether on the laboratory side in Vienna, or
on pneumothorax, x-rays or particularly in looking after TB
patients in the practice. I knew as much as anyone else of the
epidemiological aspect of the disease. On medical care, I had
had a very large and mixed practice, picking up medical skills
from my father or by myself. This was of importance, since
the overall success of a health service depends far more on the
general practitioners than on heart surgery, skyscraper hospitals or idiosyncratic ministers of health. There was a lot
more. I had for instance developed survey techniques which
could be used to solve health problems. I knew something
about nutrition and had socio-economic knowledge relating
health to poverty, disease to unemployment and to the care
of people who could not cope with living. I was influenced
by the concept of humanising medicine rather than the solely
scientific, administrative or political approaches. I had been
at the receiving end of the attention and harassment from the
Ministry of Health in the North of Ireland, I was a good union
man and had held senior posts in the British Medical Associ-

ation. So I decided to go through with it. I did so, not because
I wanted a nine-to-five job and no night calls, but because I
really wanted it as a chance to 'do things'.

Analyse it whatever way you like, there I was sitting at my
desk on the morning of 1 October 1944, ready for business.
There was a great heap of files before me, which I viewed with
suspicion and, apart from an attractive young lady secretary
who fluttered in and out, I was alone for the morning and
indeed for the next few days.

One afternoon I was invited to visit the Secretary of the
Department, Mr James Hurson. He was nice, but was visibly
upset when I asked him if I could have the terms of reference
of my post and a definition of my duties. In nineteen years I
never received either. The job was more or less what the name
implied, Chief Medical Adviser. With my staff, I was responsible for all medical advice needed in the Department: this
also included all medical inspections of the health services
and anything and everything for which technical advice and
guidance was needed. The job was both what you made it and
what you were allowed to make it. Above you was the Minister,
the political head of the Department, and the Secretary, the
administrative head who as the Accounting Officer had responsibilities of his own, even outside those of the Minister.
So far as the technical medical side of the Department was
concerned, I was the head.

Through the collective responsibility of the Cabinet the
Minister was responsible to the Dáil and was responsible for
policy and for the working of his Department. The Secretary
was responsible to the Minister for the implementation of
policy and for running the Department and to the Controller
and Auditor General as Accounting Officer. I was responsible
for the medical advice and the medical supervision of the services and through the Secretary to the Minister.

Each one was looking over his shoulder. The Minister had
to worry about the party and the voters and, of course, there
were usually powerful medical interests in the party. The
Secretary was the bureaucrat and had to ensure that the chain
of command functioned smoothly. He had also to worry
about the Department of Finance and the Controller and
Auditor General and to please the Minister. The medical staff

were mere advisers, outside the chain of command. We could not even write a letter unless expressly instructed to do so. We gave advice, knowing that the Minister was besieged by party people, who also advised behind the scenes and had political power which we did not possess. In some sectors the Secretary could more or less do as he liked. Neither need take the technical advice if they did not want to. However you could always hang it around their necks and make them responsible if anything went wrong.

In a technical area like Public Health this set-up was sheer nonsense. It meant that politics and bureaucratic power and finance could count for more than preventing disease or curing the sick. Of course no one spelt all this out to me, so I had to learn it the hard way. When the senior men or women were tolerant, intelligent and respected one another and worked together as a team, the system could be got to function. But if anyone of the 'troika' went off the rails it would eventually hit the buffers. This mixture of metaphors gives the picture of the situation which existed in practically every health department in every country which inherited the British system and which had not changed it.

After a day or so, Mr Hurson, the Secretary, brought me in to meet Dr Ward, the Parliamentary Secretary with responsibility for health matters. I had only a vague idea of who or what he was until I met him. Then it appeared that he had been a general practitioner from Monaghan town. We had worked only thirty or forty miles away from one another, but we had never met. He had gained prominence serving in the IRA during the War of Independence, then had gone into politics through membership of the Fianna Fáil party and in 1932 had been appointed to junior ministerial office. In early 1944 the Government had formally delegated to him responsibility for health, public assistance and national insurance. He was not, however, a member of the cabinet.

We soon found a common interest, which was to create a good and effective health service. He had no money or power, save what his chief could secure from the cabinet. However, there did seem to be something on the horizon with the success of the Irish Hospital Sweepstakes, the national lottery of the day designed to provide funds for health care institutions, which had provided a lot of money in the 1930s, and once the war ended would hopefully do so again. Ward had lots of ambition and was an able man but did not suffer fools and had a temper. I found that he was a good and concerned doctor in practice, but in power he had managed to antagonise the medical profession.

As it was of importance to me, I tried to analyse the factors involved. As a general practitioner he was resented by the consultants, who at that time were an arrogant lot anyway. In addition many of the consultants supported the Fine Gael party and it was the business of the opposition to defame and disparage him, and this they did with enthusiasm. People, who were sufficiently privileged to always expect to get their own way, were annoyed because he was tough enough to stand up to them and say, no! Again, in those days clever, determined people who knew their job were generally disliked in Ireland. My colleagues on the medical side in the Department later warned me over and over again not to trust Ward, and the same advice came to me from people outside. On the other hand his ideals and mine were close and in spite of his difficult manner and our odd quarrels, I liked the man.

After Dr Ward, I met Mr MacEntee, the Minister of Local Government and Public Health. I had not come across him before, although he came from Belfast. I knew his brother, who was an excellent doctor in the city and had even met his mother and sister at Lough Derg years before, without in any way connecting them with their distinguished relative. He was a most unusual product of the North of Ireland. He was a little gentleman, most cultured and courteous. Then he had a sense of humour, a biting tongue and was enormously capable. He could master a brief in a few minutes, could plan in a comprehensive way and was the epitome of the cultured European politician, something which I had never seen before from the North of Ireland. He would have been a great success in the EEC. He was also as vain as a peacock. He had a marked commonsense, was politically very able and had an immediate grasp of what the public would 'buy'. Finally, he could be pretty ruthless and I, for one, kept my distance from him. I found that I could argue without any trouble with Ward, but not with MacEntee, although others could handle him easily.

There was a reason. Ward and I spoke the same medical language and had the same interest in a problem. With MacEntee
it was different. Like all politicians, as I later found out, he
spoke a different dialect and had a different understanding
of a problem. When you introduced a purely medical situation
and explained it to him as such, he could not be got to see it
any way save in a political sense or in its political implications.
As a politician his approach was almost exclusively political,
whether government, party, public or personal. It was not so
in any cheap vote-getting sense and one had to admire him
for his wisdom, practicality and indeed courage. Sometimes it
was of supreme importance to know whether a thing was politically feasible, and if he could sell it to the cabinet, to the
party or the public. On such matters he was superb. At other
times this political approach was a nuisance so far as technical
matters were concerned. It was also important to keep him
from going off at half-cock on some health crusade or other,
a common fault with Ministers of Health everywhere.

James Hurson, the Secretary, was an elderly bachelor and a
good survivor. He never said 'yes' and never said 'no'. He was
however a good ally of mine and kept me from making a bigger
fool of myself than was strictly necessary. There were others
whom I remember, such as John Collins, a delightful official
of the old school with a wonderful sense of humour, a complete integrity and with very great ability. I also had as mentor
Tom McArdle, a Monaghan man, an Assistant Secretary, who
on the day that all officials were required to take an oath of
allegiance to the Crown, following the uprising of 1916,
walked out into what amounted to oblivion for a civil servant
rather than compromise his principles. John Garvin was a
special friend and together we would discuss the affairs of the
nation. He was one of a group of remarkable young civil servants which included Dan O'Donovan, a brilliant man who
had later a stormy career; Brian O'Nolan (otherwise Flann
O'Brien and/or Myles na gCopaleen), a Tyrone character who
was even then, without anyone appreciating it, laying the
foundations of a world reputation for his writings; and Tom
Barrington and Des Roche, who have been my friends for
more than forty years. They were a new wave of cultured
intellectuals, sophisticates who discoursed on philosophy and

literature, whether Proust, Spengler, Joyce, Sartre or Maritain or the current interest of the day. They were a most delightful, elegant lot, (elegant at least intellectually) and one could enjoy their company. I had to make the little bit of reading I had done from the Linenhall library stock go a long way with that lot.

The medical people I did not meet for a few weeks, apart from my deputy, Dr Winslow Sterling Berry. They had retired to a room somewhere up in the roof of the Custom House and decided to boycott me because I had been appointed from outside. Berry was an old 'pet'. He was the son of the Bishop of Killaloe and had been a Colonel in the RAMC, was the receptacle of all the local government and public health lore in Ireland and was very good at his work. He taught me my job, in that until I entered the Custom House I had never handled a file in my life. He showed me how to find my way around the bureaucratic maze, how to say 'yes' without committing oneself or meaning it and how to say 'no' without giving offence or meaning it as well; how to provide oneself with an escape loophole and how to 'pass the buck', because one must remember that inevitably either the politicians or the administrators would let you down.

Eventually, being decent, intelligent men and having made their protest, the medical staff sent down J.D. MacCormack to see what I was like. We spent an afternoon together talking about anything and everything and struck up a friendship which lasted for many years till he died. To me, coming from the North, he was something unusual. I had never met anyone like him. I had no idea what a tremendous person he was and how great his reputation. Whatever he said to them, the staff gradually filtered down to see me and I was able to survey my little army.

When I use the word army, it is appropriate. My predecessor, R.F. MacDonnell, was a gentleman from Roscommon, who, as a gentleman/ranker had ridden in the same troop as Winston Churchill in the last full-scale cavalry charge in modern warfare at Omdurman in the Sudan. Later he became a Colonel in the RAMC and a surgeon in the First World War and later again a Colonel in the Irish Army Medical Corps. J.D. MacCormack had earned a Military Cross in the First World War

while serving with the RAMC and had come home in a wheel-
chair, paralysed. He rehabilitated himself through golf and
was several times the Irish Amateur Champion. For years he
served on the governing body of golf at St Andrews. Professionally he was very good and had masterminded a very
successful immunisation scheme against diphtheria.

Theo MacWeeney had joined the British Army at fifteen
years of age, did his cavalry training at Ballincollig with the
Lancers, then went into the Royal Flying Corps and, when the
War was over, became the first Medical Officer of the Flight
Corps of the Irish Army. Then he went back to the RAF and
was the medical mastermind of the groups laying down land-
ing strips for the RAF route to India. He had also served for
a while in Iraq and the Persian Gulf. Paddy Ashe was a Kerry
gentleman who had been all through the First World War with
the RAMC and had been in the front line for the greater part
of his service. Charles Lysaght had been a Medical Officer in
the Irish Army and had served throughout the Civil War.

In the old troubled days, one had to be tough when carrying out some of the Department's work in Ireland. Sterling
Berry told me that when he carried out the traditional statutory inquiries into the closing of burial grounds in rural areas,
he always had a rug over his knees and under the rug a revolver.
He explained that it was sometimes necessary to wave it about
a bit to maintain order, although he had never actually fired
it. As a Protestant closing down Catholic graveyards he felt
the need for some protection. Closure of a local graveyard was
an emotional matter for country people, a kind of spiritual
and cultural eviction. It is now a forgotten experience.

Des Hourhane had not been a soldier. He was a clever, able
man and his name was plastered all over the prize boards in
the old St Vincent's hospital for the prizes and medals he had
won. Paddy Fanning was a wit and a classical scholar, the best
after-dinner speaker in Dublin, which was saying something,
and one of the best poker players in town. There was a lady,
Dr Florence Dillon, whom I did not often see. Apart from
being a Grande Dame, held in awe by the nuns everywhere,
she was one of the best bridge-players in Ireland. So this was
the team with which I started, and who for many years were
my friends. Another officer was Shane O'Neill the pharmacist,

to whom the country owes a lot.

They represented the old professional and intellectual bour-geoisie of Ireland, the mandarin class, and were a delightful, if unconscious, elite. Some of them heartily hated Ward and MacEntee and this was just as heartily reciprocated. The younger civil servants with republican backgrounds, seeing these relics of a former colonial age, with shades of the British Army, Redmondite politics and so on, did not understand them nor did they appreciate just how able they were.

Some had been 'patronage' appointments. Berry for example had been nominated for his post by Lord Carson and the Pro-testant Archbishop of Dublin, and J.D. MacCormack by his cousin John Dillon MP and by Tim Healy MP. In the old days, nominations for such posts were a valuable political perquisite and were alternated fairly evenly between the nationalist and the unionist parties. Formerly they had all been Anglo-Irish. Sterling Berry told me that when he was appointed, Sir Henry Robinson, the Vice-President of the Local Government Board, our predecessors under English rule, sent for him and said 'Dr Sterling Berry, this is a gentleman's service, keep it that way!'

MacCormack and MacWeeney took me down to Kerry on my first outing, a so-called inspection trip and the style they maintained was clear. On arrival at the hotel in Tralee, the porter rushed out, the luggage was removed and the car taken to the garage by somebody else. Meanwhile we moved in, being greeted deferentially but in a friendly way by all and sundry, were taken to a private sitting room where a good fire awaited our arrival to warm us and were then welcomed by the manager who came to discover our wishes. Later the chef came up and discussed what he should cook for us for dinner. Meanwhile the hotel porter, it was understood, cashed in on the event, by quietly visiting the hospital and various doctors to inform them of the arrival in town of the doctors from the Department.

This advance information was well used. On one visit during the trip, to the Clonakilty County Home, I was at first amazed to see that every bed seemed to have clean sheets, a clean counterpane and a clean towel. As we progressed in a stately fashion on inspection through the wards which held a very large number of beds, we were kept to a slow rate by constant introductions to staff, chit-chat from the matron and our attention being constantly drawn to this and that. In fact, as we went out of one ward, the sheets and all the rest of it were being whipped off the beds, to appear before us a bit further on. Of course you quickly knew what they were up to and you let them get away with it a few times and then exercised your intelligence and caught them out. This, if nothing else, was to let them know that the gentlemen from the Department were not complete idiots.

When the war came all routine inspections had ceased. The only car available was J.D. MacCormack's which he had solely to enable him to fight any epidemics which might occur, or to supervise the evacuation of children from Dublin, should it be necessary. The medical staff of the Department had spent the time, thus released, on special study in their various fields. MacWeeney had an hereditary interest in tuberculosis since his father had been one of the great and courageous fighters against the scourge in Ireland, so he concentrated on tuberculosis. Des Hourihan studied deafness from the public health point of view. He became so expert that some years later the US government formally requested his services as a consultant on this subject.

It is necessary to give something of the background of what we had to face and to consider the health situation in the country. For more than one hundred and fifty years under the former quasi-colonial rule, there had been a constant fight to prevent disease. From the turn of the eighteenth century Ireland had devastating epidemics of typhoid, typhus and cholera and the beginnings of the great tuberculosis epidemic which raged in the country for more than a century. There was regional over-population and the poorer the land, the more grossly over-populated it was.

Nevertheless, the long list of knights and baronets who had preceded me in my function, whatever the title, had, for over a century since the famine, tried to turn the situation around as regards public health. Within the parameters of their knowledge and the money they had to spend they had worked hard. Since the introduction of the Poor Law system they gradually created an outstanding health service by ninteenth century standards. At the turn of the century Ireland had probably the best rural health service in Europe. Our dispensary service looked after the sick poor and there was universal coverage for general practitioner care carried out by nearly a thousand doctors. The district hospitals provided hospital care throughout the country and, even though they were simply converted workhouses, they gave a good service. Though perhaps it was a bit homespun, it worked. There was a net-work of fever hospitals and emergency fever coverage and Ireland was the best vaccinated country in Europe against smallpox. We had had our last case in 1911.

Unfortunately, over several decades, the health services had ceased to progress. There were good reasons for this. One reason was that many serious disease problems were not overcome either because there was insufficient knowledge or not enough enterprise to try to eradicate them. Secondly the service was mainly based on the Poor Law, a service for indigent people, 'who through their own industry were not able to provide for themselves'. While it may have been good enough for starving people during the Famine and thereafter, it was certainly not good enough for a people better educated and more conscious of their human dignity. The public had come to hate it. The third factor was that commencing with the First World War through the War of Independence, the Civil War, the slump, the economic war, to the Second World War, the country had never known what it was to have a settled quiet period. Finally we were in a transition from a colonial regime to that of an independent country with little wealth, and in the foundation of the state and its subsequent development health had to take its place in the sharing-out of scarce national resources.

So I found myself confronted with a crumbling neglected Poor Law system which had been very badly run-down. We had the worst tuberculosis problem in Western Europe, the last louse-borne typhus in Western Europe, a chronic typhoid problem, a very high infant mortality rate with a huge number of babies dying from enteritis, a high maternal mortality rate, workhouse hospitals, few medical specialists outside of Dublin, decaying dispensaries, low standards and the senior medical establishment more concerned with sport, gracious living and

style than professional excellence. As the playboy genius
Gogarty put it, 'a doctor had first of all to be a gentleman.
After that he could be qualified.' And of course there was a
war on. The medical profession was in constant conflict with
the Department of Local Government and Public Health. With
independence, the Free State had become inward looking and
preoccupied with its own small local concerns and problems
and constrained by parochial resources.

Now for the good news. The political heads in the Custom
House and indeed the government as a whole appreciated that
things were bad and they were determined to do something
about the situation. A few years after the establishment of
the state, the Rockefeller Foundation had given £80,000, a
very large sum in those days (though much less than the Hospital Sweepstakes was to provide every year from 1930 on-
wards), to set up four experimental public health units at the
county level. This project had been a success and each county
now had a public health operation with an active well-trained
public health officer known as the County Medical Officer
of Health (CMO). They were carrying out a good schools
medical service, had already an excellent diphtheria immunisation scheme and were undertaking the tuberculosis service.
These CMOs were a competent group, just waiting to be really
used to their full capacity. We were fortunate that we had a
complete cadre of first-class general practitioners and the personnel in some other parts of the public health service were
very good indeed. My concern at the outset was with the service to the public.

The public at large were fed up with the old Poor Law system
and were scared of tuberculosis. They were demanding changes.
The medical profession were loud in their demand for improvement. Other things counted too; the Hospital Sweepstakes had
been organised since 1930 and had produced manna from
heaven. Since the 'Sweep' was illegal in both the US and Britain
receipts dropped drastically during the war, partly as a result
of postal censorship. The flow picked up again in the late
1940s but not on the scale of the 1930s. The spending of the
aforesaid manna had been controlled by the Hospitals Commission and the Hospitals Trust Fund, set up as independent
bodies to regulate the expenditure but which by judicious

manipulation had come to be very much an extension of the Custom House. A hospital building programme had been started and more than forty hospitals had been built. The Medical Research Council was functioning well. There was a galaxy of new talent coming on stream from the medical schools. These young people were likely to go abroad for further training once the war was over and we would have these as well as the large number of medical people who would hopefully return to Ireland once their service was terminated. We had the Local and Civil Service Commissioners and the Appointments Commission to enable us to secure the best candidates on a merit basis. A final factor was the ruthless determination of all the national leaders to create a new state. These people had seen the insides of gaols, some had been condemned to death and they had fought for this opportunity and nothing was going to stop them.

The system in the Custom House was not particularly conducive to action. There was a constant and steady stream of files crossing my desk, each of which had to be examined and dealt with. These came every day and all day. From the tip of Malin Head in Donegal down to Mizen at the other end of the country, every little tittle-tattle of administration required departmental approval. The file was sent to you 'to see' or 'for comment'. You in turn sent it to the Medical Inspector for the area for his comments or for him 'to see'. He then wrote something on it and sent it back and if you agreed with his views you said so, or you might send it back to him with the note 'please speak', in which case you wanted a word with him about it. Eventually it found its way back to the administrative section dealing with it and if they were not clear or satisfied it might come back again for more comment or for the Inspector to study or investigate when next in the area. When the administrative section had seen it they usually sent it up the line and it might end on the Minister's desk, or indeed the Secretary of the Department might send it back with further queries. And so the process went on.

If the Matron of a small district hospital wished to put a bottle of tomato sauce on the table for her patients, she had to go through an administrative procedure. First she had to requisition it from her store and enter it into the day-book. It then went into a weekly book and very possibly a monthly book as well. Certainly it figured in a year book and was finally featured in the annual returns. After all that the Local Government Auditor would spend quite a while perhaps trying to find out why it had never been booked into the store in the first instance or whatever. With this kind of endeavour the Local Government Audits could be many years in arrears.

One could write a book on the operation of this system. A file could be 'lost'. It might be at the bottom of the heap on someone's desk. It might remain there because he was 'out sick', or because he was a 'bottle-neck', not through his own fault but because the area for which he was responsible was jammed with activity and he had not been reinforced and could not cope. Perhaps someone who wanted to obstruct a proposal might decide to let a file roost quietly in a drawer, hoping that everyone would forget about it. It was possible to control the progress of a file by reference to the date on which someone received it and the date on which it was discharged by that person, but this technique could be obviated by sending it sideways for examination and re-examination and so on.

In theory, in a well-run department files should arrive, be examined quickly and objectively, be dealt with and despatched. They should only go to people concerned and competent to deal with them who not only knew the Minister's policy but had the technical, financial or administrative ability to handle them. But if a senior official was unable to delegate and wished to study every file scrupulously, then he would slow up the work and half the files in the department might remain 'stuck' in his room. If he was sufficiently senior, people would simply be afraid to do anything about it. If he was 'out sick' for a couple of weeks he was likely to find his office empty on his return. His juniors would have gone in, cleared the files and sent them on their way.

If you had an important project on hand it was up to you to 'chase' the file along, lest it should go to sleep on the way. You could cut corners, but no one liked it and it wasn't fair. In the Department of Health people liked one another, had common aims and wanted to get the job done, which is why we got so much done for so long. But it was a vulnerable, unsatisfactory system. In fact it was a rotten system.

Finding that Dr Sterling Berry liked 'doing' the files, was very good at it and was meticulous in spotting irregularities and correcting them, and always observed the protocol and etiquette in pushing the files around, I left him to it. Sterling Berry was so honest as to be almost naive. He liked to impress his personality on the files by always writing in green ink.

This back-up by Sterling Berry, until his retirement in 1946, was invaluable. I knew that he would keep the medical side of the Department protected, that nothing would go astray and that he would show me anything I should see. I was thus able to get on with my priorities. The problems were so urgent and the war-time conditions so difficult that it was impossible for me to just sit there and contemplate the situation making reasoned and leisurely judgements on what was to be done. I had to get out and get on with the job.

Typhus
Ireland was the last country in Western Europe with louse-borne typhus and the Anglo-Irish health administration had never mastered the disease. It came from social conditions which in parts of the country had altered very little in the previous hundred years. During the war it became a major concern to the British since, if it had made its way to the other island and they had a really bad outbreak, it could have lost the war for them. The opposite was also true: we received a tremendous plague of scabies from Britain, which kept the Irish people scratching and miserable for a couple of years till we managed to clear it up.

Therefore it was imperative that people who had a louse infestation (as so many had during the war) and who were possibly carrying the rickettsia of typhus should not travel across the water. Accordingly a Health Embarkation Scheme was set up to de-louse all those who were going to Britain to join the armed forces or to take up employment. It was a fairly hush-hush affair and people did not talk much about it lest national feelings should be hurt.

After my early talks with Dr Ward it was plain that, to clear up infectious diseases including typhus, we needed extra legal powers. Mr MacEntee agreed to put a Health Bill through the

Dáil. Unfortunately, before we had even started, it appeared in Cabinet that the Minister for Finance and his Department were against our spending any more money.

One day in November 1944 J.D. MacCormack who was responsible for infectious diseases and whose particular pet was the Health Embarkation Scheme said to me, 'I've just got word about something and you are to come to dinner tonight. I'm arranging the show and Hurson is host. MacElligott, the Secretary of Finance, is coming and Ferguson, the Secretary of Industry and Commerce. I will pick you up.'

We went first to the Globe Hotel in Talbot Street where there was quite a crowd of people milling around trying to make their way into the hotel. We pushed our way in and saw that in various rooms doctors in white coats were examining the people for lice. This was the Health Embarkation Scheme in operation. From the Globe Hotel we went to the Iveagh Baths. There I saw something I will not forget. The baths had been emptied. On the floor of a pool were large sherry half-casks. Men with rubber aprons and wellington boots were hosing people down and bathing them with disinfectant in the casks. All around were naked men, seemingly in hundreds. The place was full of steam and the smell of disinfectants.

Now naked men en masse are not a pretty sight and the atmosphere of shame, fear and outrage was easy to feel. There was a little hut in the corner where axillary and pubic hair was being shaved off and mercuric ointment rubbed in. J.D. prided himself on the thoroughness of his operation and took Mac-Elligott along to a place where a fellow with an electric iron was killing the lice in cap-bands and braces since steam disinfection, which the clothes were receiving, would perish leather and rubber. MacElligott, a man with proper susceptibilities, promptly came over faint and had to be taken outside and revived in the fresh air. Then we adjoined to the Dolphin for a good dinner. I can still remember a lobster dish served in little ramekins and the wonderful Dolphin steaks.

The next morning James Hurson brought me to the Department of Finance where we made our case for the money for the Bill to MacElligott and his colleagues. However we did not need to do any arguing or pleading since MacElligott did it for us against his own people and we got our money.

It was very difficult to know what the real typhus situation was and how widespread was the possible infection or the likelihood of a major outbreak of the disease. So, after a bit of thought, I arranged for J.D. to have blood samples taken from men passing through his scheme. This was of course quite illegal and we were probably committing common assault. We found that starting over on the west coast, where typhus was thought to be endemic, the anti-bodies in the blood against the disease were high and gradually fell for those people whose residences were near Dublin. The 'spread' of the investigation and the level of the anti-bodies found provided plenty of evidence that we had far more typhus than was thought and that a lot of people particularly in the west must have had a mild typhus subclinical attack, which may have been mistaken for influenza or other febrile illness.

Although it had been 'contained' over the years by the prompt actions of the medical staff of the Customs House, typhus had never been eradicated. The actions had sometimes been pretty ruthless and very often illegal. The new County Medical Officers were a help but not effective against the disease. There was the classic situation in the west of an impoverished population, extensive louse infestation and the presence of rickettsia. This mixture could easily blow up, get out of hand and cause a serious epidemic. The fact that one had not occurred in recent times was a matter of good fortune. This louse situation was a country-wide problem, since in the poorer industrial areas of the North of Ireland there was plenty of infestation. Just at that time DDT was introduced as a pesticide and tried out by the Allied forces in Naples. I knew the formula from my previous existence as Chemical Warfare Officer in Lurgan and I thought we should have a shot at making it ourselves. I found that a man called Donny Coyle had a small chemical manufacturing plant in Galway called Hygeia and a clever chemist Pat Moynihan.

When I went to see Hygeia I found that they were in an old warehouse at Nun's Island in Galway. While the set-up was not very impressive the two principals were. David Donovan Coyle was a Derryman who had settled in Galway. He was just about the brightest character one could hope to meet. He was clever, determined, an amazing worker, adventurous and at the same time a thoroughly decent and honest man. Pat Moynihan was a Kerryman, a brilliant chemist, a scholar, a native Irish speaker and a patriot.

I rolled out the formula, hoping to impress them with my science. It's worth writing it down since it sounds almost poetic. Dichlorodiphenolthrichlorethylene. I asked them if they could make it and Pat promptly replied that the basics were alcohol, benzine and chlorine and that was all right. Donny said that he was a director of Galway gas works and could get benzine and that there was a potato alcohol factory not too far away, and there was some question of smuggling chlorine from the North, so that was that. Anyway, I told them to go ahead and when they had made some we could test it. Later on I found out how difficult was the task that I had set them and how great their achievement was in making it. Apart from anything else I could not give them a contract and they had to trust me that they would be paid.

The alcohol and benzine had to be chlorinated separately using hydrochloric acid. With their simple apparatus there was a constant problem of chlorine gas and they had to use gas masks. Then the benzine was so impure that they had to distil it. This they did in steel containers heated over gas rings. Now to distil benzine in steel containers over gas rings was probably one of the most foolhardy and dangerous things that one could do. Apart from blowing themselves up they might well have taken half of Galway with them.

Then the chlorinated benzine had to be taken a stage further in the presence of the very concentrated sulphuric acid and this posed another problem. The reactors and the effluent were so corrosive that no metal could stand them; they also ate concrete at such a rate that there were local road subsidences and a serious difficulty in disposing of the stuff. There was the risk of the hydrochloric acid finding its way into the Galway water system and so on. When they used powdered limestone to neutralise the material they had the problem of disposing of that too.

Eventually Donny found some perfectly good ceramic apparatus lying derelict in Kynoch's old First World War munition factory in Arklow and that helped a lot. A 'tiny' explosion took the skin off Donny's face, mercifully sparing his eyes. He had to wear a beard for some time until it healed. (On one occasion, when he attended an important funeral somewhere, wearing mourning dress, the local paper commented on the unexpected arrival of the Chief Rabbi at the obsequies.)

Once they got going, they produced about ten tons of DDT a year. This was mixed with talc from the Donegal barytes mine to make a five per cent mixture, so that we had a yearly output of two hundred tons of DDT.

J.D. MacCormack insisted on testing the first batch of DDT himself. The rest of us were married with children and so he must be the one. He went around with watch-glasses strapped to his arms and abdomen and under these were lice and different concentrations of our homemade DDT. Of course he could have caught typhus if some of the lice had rickettsia and the so-called DDT hadn't worked. He stayed on this until he found the concentrations which gave the quickest 'kill' of the lice. His descriptions of the 'dance of death' of the lice were macabre. He soon became an authority on lice and his lectures to various medical societies, in which he would explain the sex habits of the louse, were hilarious. One Saturday morning he said that he would carry out his final test, but would not tell me what it was. In fact he ate five grammes of the stuff and then played thirty-six holes of golf at Portmarnock.

He came in to the office on Monday morning none the worse for his experiment save that he had great haematomata on his hands where the DDT, the golf clubs and J.D.'s proverbial long hitting had caused haemorrhages under the skin. He then pronounced that our DDT was safe and would not poison children. However I wanted to try it out a bit further before, so to speak, 'going public'. Talking it over with some of the County Medical Officers, Dr Bill MacCarthy of Kildare told me that they were having a serious problem of lice and flea infestation in the turf camps. During the war, there was little or no imported fuel available and so a great emergency programme of digging turf (peat) was organised. Large numbers of men were concentrated on the bogs and were housed in whatever accommodation could be found under emergency conditions. With Bill MacCarthy, J.D. and I went down to Edenderry where a number of turf-diggers were housed in the old workhouse. There we met the medical officer in charge, Dr Tom Murphy. He gave us a demonstration of his problem and we decided to help. J.D. took on the job of providing supplies of DDT and of giving guidance on how it was to be used. The success of the trial was due to Tom Murphy, who later became President of UCD. He had worked hard on the problem, had developed a mobile delousing unit and had done everything possible under very difficult conditions but without being able to clear it up. However the DDT in his hands worked wonders. We distributed it free through the local dispensaries and other channels such as schools. During those difficult times Ireland was the first country to have everywhere available the very great boon of pesticide and in this way, freedom from lice, fleas and bugs.

Of course the Department's medical officers were not the only people concerned. The success of the whole project in the country depended on the County Medical Officers. They became enthusiastic in the campaign to eradicate typhus, breaking the chain of transmission of the disease by eradicating lice, the carriers of the rickettsia.

Accordingly they moved in with DDT where the problem was greatest, such as in the villages and the isolated houses on the more remote parts of the Atlantic seaboard. There they made sure that every house was plastered with the stuff and that the lice problem was finished. Sometimes this was resented, and I have to record that the late Dr Charles MacConn, CMO for Galway, received a crack over the head with an iron bar for his enthusiastic pursuit of rickettsia-bearing lice.

One day while this was going on a gentleman came into my office and said that he understood that we were making DDT. He said he represented Geigy, who held the world patents covering the manufacture of this material and that we would have to stop making it. I put him off and arranged a later meeting. When he had gone I rang Donny Coyle in Galway. He found from his patent agent that when the Free State was established, somehow or other Geigy had failed to cover themselves in this country. When Geigy's represetnative returned he was told this and that we were going to continue to make it and would soon start to export. This was of course more or less a joke. Immediately a delegation arrived from Manchester, where Geigy had a factory, and an instant offer was made to Donny followed by an agreement. If we had not been free to make it, they might have stopped us.

DDT was also welcome in schools where head-lice had become a problem which had intensified with the war. Few realise to-day the difficulties the poor and those with large families had in procuring soap and heating water to maintain cleanliness, particularly amongst children. Anyway, we have not had a case of typhus since.

Donny and Pat made other contributions in the Emergency period. When de Valera told the Irish farmers to plough up their land and grow wheat during the war he did not reckon with rhincosporum or blackspot. In consequence the yield of wheat was greatly reduced and without a mercuric fungicide would have become less each successive year. Fungicide to spray and protect the wheat could not be obtained. Commodore Poole, my neighbour and friend in Wexford, told me that he brought in five tons of mercury from Spain in one of Stafford's little ships sailing out of Wexford. It was a very dangerous war-time voyage for a neutral and he was lucky to get home afloat, having been attacked. The mercury was taken to Donny and Pat Moynihan in Galway and they made enough ethyl mercuric chloride to protect the Irish wheat crop. Once they had made it, supplies of fungicide immediately became available from ICI at a very low price. Donny also made ordinary domestic disinfectant, which was not available here in war-time, and chlorinated phenol for sheep-dip. Without sheep-dip a flock of sheep can become infested with maggots in literally a few hours and it becomes a miserable and difficult job to get them clear again; meanwhile the animals suffer badly.

Donny had water-rights and a turbine at Coloony in Sligo and made carbide. Without carbide at that time no welding could have been done in the country. I mention these things to show how a small neutral country can be vulnerable in unexpected ways in war-time.

Early Days in the Custom House

The fact that 'there was a war on' was an excuse for every lazy, incompetent character. The effect of such an attitude could be terrible. I can remember going into a ward in some small TB place in Limerick and seeing a young girl sitting up in bed and looking sadly at her dinner plate which was on her bed without even a tray. She was near to death and, apart from the damage to her lungs, had tuberculous laryngitis and could only speak in whispers. She could hardly swallow. On her plate was a piece of burnt steak, a spoonful of cabbage and two blackened potatoes. I flew into a rage with the matron who confessed that she was unable to give her cornflour, rice or some milk dish that she could swallow because it was not allowed on the instructions of some administrator. Later I went to see him and he pleaded ignorance of anything that went on in the institution which he rarely visited because of his fear of infection.

The doctor in charge of the place was as bad and when MacWeeney and I had finished with him he resigned. All in a good cause but of course quite illegal and to-day we would never get away with it. Limerick generally was very bad. They had some kind of maternity and child welfare set-up in a place called Bedford Row. It was dirty and seemed to be used very seldom. I found the dried slime of snail-tracks on the examination couches.

When inspecting the City Home and Hospital the matron, an elderly nun, every few paces lamented the good old days when the doctors from the Department were gentlemen. Everything that was not in a ward was locked up and she could not find the keys. But I waited until they were eventually procured. When the doors were finally opened they revealed in several ground floor compartments some beautiful young yearling racehorses belonging to the medical officer who was a decent man and a powerful political figure. The older inmates, who were expert with horses, exercised them for him. When I got down to basics the inmates told me that these horses were the most important thing in their lives and to take them away would break their hearts. So I left them there — the place was a shambles anyway.

Limerick as a city needed a central health clinic, but the officials always said that they could not find a suitable premises. I went down and found one in a single morning. The fact was that they did not want any disturbance.

One of the things I tried to do was to organise public health monitoring. For example, going through returns for infant deaths in Cork I noticed that there was something unusual and traced the matter to a home for unmarried mothers at Bessborough outside the city. I found that in the previous year some 180 babies had been born there and that considerably more than 100 had died. Shortly afterwards, when in Cork, I went to Bessborough. It was a beautiful institution, built on to a lovely old house just before the war, and seemed to be well-run and spotlessly clean. I marched up and down and around about and could not make out what was wrong; at last I took a notion and stripped all the babies and, unusually for a Chief Medical Adviser, examined them. Every baby had some purulent infection of the skin and all had green diaorrhoea, carefully covered up. There was obviously a staphylococcus infection about. Without any legal authority I closed the place down and sacked the matron, a nun, and also got rid of the medical officer. The deaths had been going on for years. They had done nothing about it, had accepted the situation and were quite complacent about it.

A couple of days later I had a visit in Dublin from the nuns' 'man of affairs' and he was followed by the Dean of Cork, Monsignor Sexton, and finally the Bishop of Cork complained to the Nuncio, who went to see de Valera. The Nuncio, Archbishop Robinson, (formerly a millionaire American stockbroker) saw my report and said we were quite right in our action. For once the Bishop, Dr Lucey, a formidable fighting man, was silent.

Later, when the place had been disinfected and repainted and so on, the Order supplied a new matron and we appointed a new doctor. During the succeeding years, while many hundreds of babies were born each year, the number of deaths never exceeded single figures. To-day the deaths of only a few infants in such an institution will bring about a furore in the press.

Dr Ita Brady, the schools' medical officer for County Dublin came to see me one day in the Custom House. She said that the primary schools in the county were in a shocking state, that no one would do anything about it and that she was fed up. I went out with her the next day and we spent the morning and afternoon looking at them. We took a camera along and took photographs of the worst of them. Ita Brady was quite right, the situation was dreadful.

Dirt, overcrowding, dilapidation and lack of simple hygiene were so bad as to be a serious threat to the health of the children. I remember that in Balrothery national school a window was broken. Someone had taken the seat off a lavatory to close the gap and to close the hole in the seat had cleverly filled it in with an atlas stuck down with drawing pins. The report I made found its way on to Mr de Valera's desk and he sent it to Dr MacQuaid, the Archbishop of Dublin, since the schools were run by the clergy. One of the worst of the schools was only a stone's throw from MacQuaid's house at Killiney. I am afraid that we rather highlighted that one. MacQuaid reacted badly to the report and that started another row. In one sense it was unfair to blame him. The local authority, the Department of Education and their Schools Inspectors, the Office of Public Works, the teachers, the parents of the children, all were involved. This report began a clean-up of the schools. It paved the way, by its being accepted as a priority, for a great schools building programme.

One problem we were early faced with was the famous Fever Hospital in Cork Street, Dublin. It had been founded and conducted by the Quakers for more than one hundred years. But, as in all these elderly institutions, the funds were beginning to dry up and the Board of Governors appealed to the government to bail them out. The buildings were a bit antiquated and the Board had decided to build a new hospital and had secured a site at Cherry Orchard, outside the city. The plans on the architects' drawing board were to say the least of it somewhat elaborate, reflecting the thinking of Dr Chris MacSweeney, the medical superintendent, a distinguished fever expert. I remember they proposed a nine hole golf links in the grounds for the staff, some of whom liked golf.

The government, that is to say, Mr MacEntee and Dr Ward, took the opportunity to reconstitute the Board. With the Quakers, the original owners, they included representatives of the Dublin Corporation and the Dublin County Council and, to make the mix interesting, two specially nominated representatives of the Minister of Local Government and Public Health. That gave four special interests, all of whom were concerned with the running of the Hospital. One might even include Chris MacSweeney the Superintendent, as a fifth. It seemed a very reasonable way to approach the future hospital provision for infectious diseases for the city and county of Dublin. Extraordinarily, this mixture provided the contestants for one of the most prolonged and bitterly fought battles that had been seen in Ireland since the Civil War. The rows raged, blazed and spilled out from the boardroom of the hospital all over the town. The press got a hold of it and wrote it up extensively, and eventually the Minister's two representatives appealed to him to do something. Mr MacEntee ordered a sworn Inquiry and J.D. MacCormack was given the task of conducting it.

J.D. took it very seriously and went out and bought a new outfit, including an Anthony Eden hat, so as to give himself a 'Kings Inns' appearance and impress the bevy of lawyers employed by the various sides. Unfortunately, he was in a 'no win' situation; he might as well have put his hand into a bagfull of ferrets. No matter how he questioned the witnesses or treated them (and J.D. was always most courteous) they all thought that he was against them and favouring the other parties. The newspapers went to town in writing up the Inquiry and were inclined to slant it one way or another as they too took sides. MacEntee got very annoyed that it was not going his way and the whole thing was as big a mess at the end as it was in the beginning. My colleagues tried to keep me out of it since they thought that I was too young and innocent.

However, it was not easy. For example, an old friend would invite me to dinner at some such place as the United Services Club and when the dinner was nearing its end, a group dining at a neighbouring table who were known to my friend would find their way over and join us. I would find that I was the target for a carefully contrived bit of lobbying as all the people there were up to their eyes in the business. This kind of thing one could take in one's stride and really it meant nothing, but eventually it turned vicious.

My Strike
While I was, so to speak, playing myself in, familiarising myself with the problems, getting to know people and dealing as

best I could with the more glaring defects, I came up against
authority. Dr Ward became fed up with my wandering around
the country and not being available when he needed me. De
Valera had sent for him and asked him questions about something with which I had been concerned and he quite reasonably
hadn't the answers, but he had been embarrassed. He gave me
an instruction that I was to have clearance before going off
on my trips.

At the same time I was being manoeuvred into a false
position on semi-political things like the standards to be
adopted for blind pensions. In rural areas attempts were often
made to use these as political patronage, rather than relating
them to the capacity of people to see. Personally, I couldn't
care about such a matter, if this was the way they wanted it
so be it. There were lives to save and more important things
to do. The opposition in the Dáil should deal with any such
irregularities. But I had an Ophthalmic Inspector on the staff
of the Department, Dr Fleming, an honest man who took his
job very seriously. He was responsible for certifying whether
people would qualify for such pensions and he was fed up
with political interference from all sides; of course I supported
him. I told Dr Ward to leave us alone and if the politicians in
the Dáil wanted anything different they should change the
Act, which of course I knew they would not do.

Finally, a political 'hack', as the man would be described
to-day, came into my office and said that the cumainn (political clubs) in the city were not pleased with the way that an
inquiry into what had gone wrong at the Cork Street Hospital
had been conducted and decided that the person involved,
J.D. MacCormack, should be dismissed. It was noticed that I
was seen to be frequently in his company and they did not
want to involve me in it in any way. So I was to avoid him in
future, as he was for the 'high jump'. I was pretty well outraged at this, so when he had gone I made a verbatim account
of the conversation, took it down to the Secretary and told
him that I had another copy. He was to show it to the Minister
and if anything happened to J.D. I would publish it.

I became increasingly unhappy about the whole situation.
My father, who had never really wanted me to leave Lurgan,
said that I would always be welcome to come home and I was

on the point of walking out and going North again. The next day, going down the Rathmines Road on the top of a tram, I saw some young women walking up and down in the rain outside a laundry, on strike. At first I pitied them because it was so wet, but then I said to myself, 'if those lassies have the courage to fight, then I must be a mouse to run away.'

At lunch that day, in the Stephen's Green Club, I let it be known gently that I was not going back to work that afternoon because I was on strike. They thought I was joking, but I was serious. After lunch, I retired upstairs to the library, where I sat it out for the next couple of days. Now the Stephen's Green Club was not only a marvellous gossip centre but a gathering place at that time for Fine Gael; in fact it was one of their 'watering-holes'. Naturally they were delighted by this chance to embarrass the government. People stuck their heads into the library to see if I was still there; considerable interest was shown in the happening.

The Secretary warned me that he would have to suspend me if I went on with this action. My medical colleagues from the Department came to visit and politely intimated that I was mad. On the third day I received a summons to attend at the Custom House. I did so and, after a blazing row with Ward and MacEntee, walked out. Eventually, peace was restored through the Secretary of the Department. One of the conditions of the peace was that I should appear in the officials' box in the Dáil when Dr Ward was introducing the Health Bill. This I did and when Dr Ward had finished his introductory speech on the Bill General Mulcahy rose and denounced him, saying that he was fighting with the Church, the medical profession and even with his own Chief Medical Adviser. Dr Ward, in replying, paid me the most handsome compliments and tributes, as had been arranged. It is all recorded in the Dáil Debates.

Chief Medical Officers, Directors of Health Services, Chief Medical Advisers, Health Commissioners or Vice-Ministers of Health or whatever their title or function, all over the world have been imprisoned, exiled, executed or just sacked. They have been made the scapegoats for their political masters and suffered or resigned or even in despair have sought the support of their professional colleagues. But so far as I know, I am the only one to have had the guts, folly or impertinence to go on strike and get away with it. But actually it was all due to the little laundry girls. This daft impulse had the effect that from now on, I was my own master!

Conditions started to ease a bit in 1945; the Inspectors started on the road again and became busy; and the political and administrative people were occupied with the Health Bill, so I did two studies. The first, on typhoid, was a fairly straightforward affair, the second, on enteritis, was more difficult.

Typhoid

Throughout the country there had been on average about 350 confirmed cases of typhoid a year during the ten years from 1935 to 1945, and usually about fifty deaths. This despite a very comprehensive network of fever hospitals, disinfection stations, the availability of anti-typhoid inoculations and a keenly active County Public Health Organisation. In addition there were more and more piped water supplies and proper sewage installations. Outbreaks were usually rapidly controlled but they kept recurring.

With the help of the County Medical Officers, I collected all the records on 1,000 cases and analysed them. I set down about eighty questions that we should try to answer. Although the cases and outbreaks were scattered they showed a fairly consistent pattern. In particular it appeared that more than 60 per cent of all cases came from houses where there had been typhoid within the previous fifteen years.

We sent each County Medical Officer a list of all the reported cases of typhoid which had occurred in his county within the previous fifteen years. They organised visits to the houses and collected samples of blood, urine and faeces from all the people living in the houses, as well as immunising them with TAB vaccine. In this way we rounded up more than three hundred carriers of the disease, the vast majority of whom we had not known. Many were associated with the sale or distribution of foodstuffs. This study not only revealed the cause of the continuing small epidemics, the carriers, but indicated where and how to find them. I published a paper on the investigation in the *Irish Medical Journal* in September 1946.

The field work in the campaign was coordinated by J.D. MacCormack and later by Harry O'Flanagan. They had great fun with it, a kind of medical detective exercise. They set up a Typing Laboratory in University College Cork and were able to pin-point where any further cases came from. Occasionally the work even had an historical interest. Typhoid had been smouldering around the town of Clonmel for a long time. They were able to show that it belonged to the Truro strain, which had been brought back from the South African War by the Munster Fusiliers who had had their regimental depot in that town.

In those days there was not very much you could do about carriers, but by monitoring them and keeping them away from food-processing it was possible to maintain a lot of control. Once you knew what to do it was not too difficult. However if one County Medical Officer had fallen down on the job, the whole thing would have been a failure, for that particular area would have become a reservoir for the future spread of the disease.

As an example of what could happen, Dr Russell, CMO of Dublin City, monitoring his carriers, found that one young lady had left his area and was acting as a cook in a fashionable seaside hotel in Greystones, Co Wicklow. He rang Dr Beckett, the CMO for County Wicklow (uncle of Sam Beckett, the writer), and told him where she was. Beckett went to the hotel immediately, and, fearful lest he should have an epidemic on his hands, particularly in an hotel where a lot of children were staying, told the proprietors that she could not act as cook and she was dismissed.

A sympathetic solicitor assisted her in taking an action against poor Beckett. This was some time in 1946/47. J.D. and I went down to Wicklow to give evidence on Beckett's behalf. I saw the young lady concerned and we both felt sorry for her as she was a very pleasant, handsome young person.

Judge Maguire, who happened to be a friend of my father's, gave me a bad time in the witness box. Before I could give my evidence, he interrupted counsel who was giving an account of my importance as a witness, by asking 'what did I happen to know about typhoid?', and then giving his own view 'that I was only a civil servant from the Custom House'. From my memory, he ended up telling the jury that they should find for the plaintiff, which he hoped they would and that he hoped they would award her generous damages. In the event they gave her £600, a large sum in those days. This sort of Gilbert and Sullivan affair, coupled with the fact that we had 300 carriers that we knew of, inspired some of the tougher sections in the Health Bills we tried to get through the Dáil to protect the public.

To have such a lady, a carrier, happily cooking away in a residential hotel, full of families, knowing that she could cause an epidemic of typhoid and that you, the County Medical Officer, could be blamed, was no joke. The fact that so many CMOs went ahead anyway showed their courage, since they had little or no protection for their efforts in dealing with such cases.

From an average of 350 cases and 50 deaths a year from 1935 to 1945, we brought it down to an average of 153 cases a year and 14 deaths between 1945 and 1950. During the next five years, from 1950 to 1955, it came down to 43 cases a year and 3 deaths; by 1960, we had 10 cases and no deaths. A few years after that it had gone.

If you included the network of fever hospitals which we maintained, the tragedy of fifty preventable deaths each year, the cost of keeping 350 people in hospital for a minimum stay of six weeks, the chronic ill-health which many suffered after typhoid and the cost of the surveillance of carriers, this condition had been quite an expensive little item in the health bill of the country. Without the eradication of typhoid we could never had developed a satisfactory tourist industry. We needed to be able to guarantee that people visiting Ireland could do so without the risk of contracting the disease.

Enteritis in Infants

Between 1935 and 1941 enteritis in infants had become endemic in Ireland and five to six hundred babies died each year from this cause. Since 1941 the number had increased and 1,000 deaths occurred yearly. Of these, 600 took place in Dublin and 400 in the rest of the country. My first study defined the epidemiological problem very clearly within the limits of the knowledge available at that time.

I found that the disease mainly affected the children of poorer families, living in the poorer districts of Dublin. It was contagious and usually attacked babies in the first month of life. The study proved conclusively the epidemic nature of the disease. I collected all the known information about the disease and compared the Irish experience with that abroad. There was a lot more besides, but the important thing was that it put the whole problem in its proper perspective.

Shortly before I came to the Department, Dr Ward, in an endeavour to do something for the condition, had taken over the old Claremont Protestant Deaf and Dumb Training School and renamed it St Clare's Hospital. It was established as an isolation unit admitting only babies with enteritis. It was afterwards apparent that this was a most valuable advance.

For the second study, to define the clinical signs and symptoms of the disease, I analysed 1,604 cases admitted to this hospital. I was fortunate that the resident medical officer was Dr Dan O'Brien, a very bright young man indeed. He had been sickened by the never-ending stream of babies turning up for admission and so many dying that he was even then experimenting with rehydration methods, years ahead of his time. We found that the babies affected were mainly of low birthweight and that the disease was of sudden onset. We also established that there was a Dublin form of the disease. The overwhelming factor which seemed to influence the onset of enteritis was the failure to breast-feed the babies and the common use of cow's milk. We got a very clear picture of the disease as it affected our children and this was of value in diagnosis and the subsequent treatment.

We carried out other studies. For instance Dr Fanning studied the transmission of a possible virus cause. He worked with Pat Harnett MRCVS, who at that time was on our staff. They used calves and we organised cooperation with Michigan State University Virus Laboratory, one of the very few early virus centres. We were not able to determine a virus cause, which was not surprising considering the scanty knowledge of virology forty years ago.

I found that places like the Rotunda Hospital were foci of infection and that hospital out-patient departments, where sick children gathered, were deadly. A mother might bring a healthy child to an out-patient's department to seek help for something like a hernia and the next day the child would have enteritis, picked up at the hospital.

An interesting thing was that the Coombe Lying-in Hospital never had enteritis. There they stuck to the old-fashioned idea of putting the babies in the same beds with the mothers. This seemed to have two effects. One was that they had a higher rate of breast-feeding than the others. The other was that, not only had the babies the protection of the colostrum in the breast milk, but as their gastro-intestinal canals were invaded by bacteria in the normal way after birth these bacteria came from the mother and in some way, then unknown, conferred a degree of the mother's immune mechanism on the child.

One of our main problems was to convince the paediatricians that this was an epidemic disease. It was necessary to prevent them admitting cases to outpatients or to hospital cots. They had to be persuaded to treat infants with regard to the infectious nature of the disease. Using the criteria determined by our study, we wanted them to diagnose cases early by keeping a constant look-out for the signs and symptoms of the disease.

In fairness, this attitude was not peculiar to Dublin paediatricians. Everywhere clinical people were looking at individual cases, treating each case, trying to cure it, doing the best they could for it; seeing the problem of each child as a separate entity. Whereas we were seeing the overall problem as a serious epidemic. Whether enteritis was in Dublin, in Israel or the cities of the US, the same thing happened. One result of all this was that I was thrust into controversy with the paediatricians.

It should be understood that this problem was only one of the many for the ordinary people in the Dublin slums. They were finding it hard enough to live and all this fuss about babies was not received with any great public interest or sympathy. A baby dying here or another there was to be expected. Very few could appreciate that six hundred little Dublin souls going to heaven every year, though perhaps well out of this cruel world, was from a public health point of view something preventable, something terrible, and something to be stopped at all costs.

The fact that I did not know the cause of the disease was no excuse for doing nothing. I did know that it was contagious, that if we could prevent healthy babies being brought into contact with children with enteritis we could achieve something. So, on more or less such principles, I planned a 'cordon sanitaire' control.

People might think that to organise to cope with hundreds of infant deaths should be straightforward. In fact it was very difficult. All sorts of vested interests were involved and the in-fighting was terrific. I came in for a lot of 'stick' and abuse.

One day, for instance, I was invited to a meeting in the Children's Hospital in Harcourt Street, supposedly to discuss the situation with the paediatricians. Bob Collis, one of my friends, a paediatrician with an international reputation, a great man and one dedicated to the care of children everywhere, set out to prove that I was wrong. He showed that he had removed a child from St Clare's hospital, where he had been appointed as a consultant, and admitted it to the National Children's Hospital in Harcourt Street and that nothing had happened. I lost my temper and so far as I can recall called him irresponsible and a potential murderer.

I always found 'hard to take' the extraordinary animus against the Custom House and the people in it. It was not that we wanted to be loved, but everything we did or tried to do was met with suspicion and resistance. It was particularly noticeable in our relations with the Dublin Corporation and the Dublin 'Medical Establishment', but even bishops did not hesitate to refer to us as 'faceless civil servants'.

The doctors formed cliques fiercely loyal to their hospitals and colleagues, were closely associated with their medical schools and exercised great political and social power. The consultants treated the poor without charge in the hospitals, which really were charitable institutions. They received no salaries or stipends and lived off their private patients. In their dealings with the Department many were more than a little arrogant and often quite rude. It used to upset me when some insignificant character who had never really achieved anything and who owed his post to patronage would describe a reasonable proposition as 'another Custom House swindle'. To be patronised as a mere public health man and a civil servant was bad enough but I also was a Fellow of the Royal College of Physicians and a member of the Royal Irish Academy and had done more original things in medicine than any of them. So I am afraid that I was just as rude and scathing with some of my professional colleagues. On the other hand I had a lot of friends but they were mostly the academics and research workers as well as my own fraternity of public health men and women.

In an attempt to convince the paediatricians that enteritis was an epidemic we invited them all out to St Clare's Hospital for a conference and to see the place. They remained unconvinced and the only satisfaction I got out of it was that most of them got diaorrhoea after the visit. We appointed paediatric consultants to St Clare's thinking to soften them up and secure their cooperation and support but nothing very much came out of it.

At some medical meeting or other, possibly in the Royal Academy of Medicine, Bob Collis said that the Regina Coeli Hostel was in a terrible state, that babies were dying there and that conditions were abominable. The next morning I went along to have a look at the place. It was operated by a religious, lay, voluntary body called the Legion of Mary. The Founder was an extraordinary little man called Frank Duff. His brother was a friend of mine in the Stephen's Green Club and was the Secretary of the Department of Justice.

Frank Duff resented any interference from anybody, was bound by the rules and regulations of the Legion, which he had written himself, was a living saint, having devoted his life to this extraordinary mission. When in conversation, if he did not want to agree to anything he simply turned off his hearing aid. I managed to get in and have a good look around the place. It was very difficult to come to any conclusion on what he was doing, but he did have babies with enteritis there. After my shouting at him, he agreed to allow me to help.

Miss Howett, my wonderful secretary (afterward with WHO), organised a 'whip-around' in the Custom House and collected £25 and with this I prevailed on Frank Duff to give me a little room, which we furnished as a kind of quarantine station. The Hostel was for unmarried mothers and when one of these girls arrived with her baby to seek shelter I made the

Legionnaires put her into this little room and keep her there for five days. After this, if her baby was healthy she was allowed into the Home. In this way we gradually cleaned up the place. Once you start something you never can tell where it will end. We soon found that when babies did show green diaorrhoea or enteritis that many of them came from or had just been discharged from the Rotunda, Collis' own hospital.

When I had sorted out this information, I went to the Rotunda one morning where I found Ninian Faulkner, the Master, in bed in the Master's Lodging suffering from flu. Standing at the end of his bed I denounced him and his paediatrician Collis for spreading the disease all over the city and demanded that no child should be discharged till it had been examined, and that he should clean up the place.

I believe that Ninian Faulkner, whom I liked very much, nearly got a relapse. You could do that kind of thing in those days. People could speak their minds and remain friends with those they attacked, but whom they still respected. If I behaved today as I did then, I would be in the High Court at least once a week.

I may seem to be hard on the paediatricians, but really they were not so bad as perhaps I make out. They were a most estimable body of men and women. But all over the world, whether Dublin, New York or Israel, clinical paediatricians had one attitude towards disease in children and tried to cure it and Public Health people had another and tried to prevent it. It was like two different religions.

Dublin Corporation was even worse than the doctors. One way or another the governors of this city had had a continuity for more than 1,000 years, since the Vikings sat around the tree on the Thingmote in the present Great Andrew Street. The corporate members and their officials were immensely proud and old and wise in the ways of local government.

Dublin had appointed the first City Medical Officer in these islands and the Royal College of Surgeons of Ireland in Dublin claimed to have awarded the first Diploma in State Medicine in the world. The Corporation knew what it was doing and did not intend to have any interference from any 'upstart' government department in any new 'Free State'. On the other hand the city's public health record was terrible. At the turn of the century, Dublin had the worst slums in Europe and the greatest poverty. It was probably at its worst in the period just before the First World War and during the awful six-months general strike in 1913. The colonial neglect of Dublin had got to such a point that had there not been a political armed rebellion in Dublin in 1916, shortly after there would have been a socialist armed revolution.

During the Second World War, in spite of our being neutral, the women and children in Dublin, particularly the poor, took a tremendous beating. Wet turf with which to cook and heat, a short daily period of gas 'glimmer', shortages, deprivation and poverty. War-time for the Lurgan people was relative prosperity; for the Dublin poor, it meant that their poverty and misery grew worse.

The city had a few understaffed and poorly attended child welfare clinics and the organisation of the relatively large district nursing service was downright bad. This is not to criticise the nurses, it was the organisation, which with the war had grown slack. All over the place innovation seemed to be resented. Even the excellent maternity hospitals paid insufficient attention to neonatal deaths and the obstetricians did not welcome the paediatricians into the labour wards.

On instructions from Dr Ward and Mr MacEntee I visited Dublin City Hall on several occasions during the anti-enteritis campaign and was told not to mince words about the situation. I tried to cajole, to bully or persuade them into action without success. On one occasion I took J.D. MacCormack and somebody else from the Department as a delegation and put it up to the public health people and the City Manager that we would write out a scheme and give it to them, that they could then submit it to us and that we would approve of it and give them the money to put it into action. They simply laughed at us. It was the usual story of elderly people who had done a tremendous job in their day only to find it criticised and ridiculed by young interlopers with new ideas.

In the end Mr MacEntee, to his eternal credit, called the Public Health Committee of the Dublin Corporation into the Custom House and threatened to go to the Dáil and to have them dissolved if they did not do what they were told and carry out measures as indicated by us to try to end the situation. They were told that if they had better ideas than ours we would listen to them and let them go ahead and implement them. There was violent arguing to get it into their thick heads that we were not talking politics but trying to save babies' lives. After a lot of wrangling we established in Dublin Corporation Health Department a special unit run by Dr Paddy O'Callaghan, a Donegal genius who died young, working with Paddy Fanning from the Department. This provided for the reporting and immediate isolation of any affected child into St Clare's Hospital, disinfection of everything in the houses or tenement and a resuscitation service manned around the clock, since an hour could make all the difference between life and death for a baby with this condition. We did a lot more besides, including special attention to the quality and distribution of the milk being supplied by the Infant Aid Society, which supplied milk to poor families. We got the unit as quickly as we could into effective operation. The next year we had the deaths down from 600 to 200 and of course they fell further thereafter.

The first paper on enteritis was published in the *Journal of the Irish Medical Association* in October 1946 and the editor, Oliver Fitzgerald, wrote an editorial called 'The Lost Town' and compared the holocaust of baby deaths over five years from this one disease alone to the loss of the population of an average Irish town. The second paper, written with Dan O'Brien, was published in the same Journal in December 1946. These papers and the campaign to end the infant deaths from enteritis were highlights in the long story of my efforts to better the care and save the lives of infants and children.

Laboratory Services
I next tackled the laboratory services. Dublin had some forty medical laboratories. These ranged from little back-room affairs in small hospitals, poorly equipped and with few staff, to the larger units in University College, Trinity Medical School and the Royal College of Surgeons, which were really commercial undertakings and money spinners for the university or college concerned. The west was served by one small concern in University College, Galway, where Professor Walsh carried on the laboratory, in addition to several other respon-

sibilities including that of university bursar. He had one elderly attendant. Cork had two laboratories, one in University College, something like the Dublin units in the medical schools but much smaller. There was another in one of the many small hospitals in Cork. Some people headed up several laboratories, which they visited on a peripatetic routine. The cost of tests was far too high and the number carried out was by any standard far too low.

Paddy Fanning took, at my request, forty blood specimens in triplicate and sent them to UCD and TCD and to the RCSI laboratories, where they were tested for syphilis by the Wassermann test. From memory there was a 20 per cent plus or minus difference in the results. This of course gave a strong reason to doubt the quality and accuracy of the work. We called a meeting and invited the entire senior laboratory personnel of the country to attend. We confronted them with the Wassermann results and there was an immediate outcry at such a dirty trick of comparing the results as between one laboratory and another. I came in for a lot of 'stick' over that. In due course we invited them to discuss the rationalisation of the existing services and asked for proposals for a new service. We had no ulterior motives, had only the hope of improving the services and made no attempt at manipulation. It was a decent honest approach.

There then followed days of wrangling, defiance and 'bloody-mindedness'. They resented and distrusted the Department, did not see any sense in our trying to bring the laboratories into closer relationship with the health problems of the country, to increase the volume of work they did and to reduce the costs. They did not like a pet plan of mine, to organise a good bio-chemical service. They were annoyed at the accusation that there was very little research being done.

Today, I would handle it very differently. But forty years ago we had not the techniques for the holding of large and difficult conferences that we have now. But I was on to a loser from the beginning. Most of the people there were very senior, many had actually founded the laboratories they were running: their life-time achievements. They were well satisfied with what they had done. They felt that their livelihoods and their independence was at stake and did not see why they should cooperate, except a long way ahead and then on their own terms.

On the whole they were very intelligent people, indeed many were national figures and were very powerful politically and socially. One of them was W.D. O'Kelly, who was Professor of Bacteriology and Public Health in University College Dublin at the time of the meeting and also Bacteriological Adviser to the Department and a class-fellow of my father's. Albeit politely, he treated me as a young, impudent juvenile.

It must be appreciated that we, in this country, were no better or no worse than elsewhere. This was more or less the universal laboratory situation. In Britain they had much the same set-up till the war came and then that marvellous man G.S. Wilson went to Winston Churchill and pointed out that if they had chemical or bacterial warfare from Hitler they were completely unprepared. Churchill told him to organise whatever was needed. Wilson took advantage of this opportunity and organised the best laboratory service in the world, which has lasted ever since.

I learnt from this performance that the Dublin laboratory service would be a very hard nut to crack. The only way to do anything was to organise it from the periphery. Accordingly, as we built each of the regional hospitals we established a first class regional laboratory, linked it with the medical school so that the Professor of Pathology was also Chief of the Regional Service. In a short time we had a complete and highly efficient laboratory coverage of the country outside of Dublin.

So far as Dublin was concerned we set up a good Public Health Laboratory under Dublin Corporation with John Stritch in charge. For St James' Hospital and the other Local Authority or Municipal hospitals we organised a first-class hospital laboratory under John Harmon, then just returned from America. So the professors had a bit of competition which was good for them and more importantly benefitted the people we were all serving.

Food and Nutrition

When I came into the Custom House there was quite a lot of interest in nutrition both in the Department and outside as well. The Irish Medical Association had established a Dietetic Committee and things were happening. At this time two small surveys were carried out. They did not amount to much since they were too small to be applied nationally. But one showed very clearly that we had a serious problem of rickets in Dublin. The other created a distinct unease about the nutrition situation. However the matter had become political and the occurrence of a death in Allihies in West Cork, believed to be due to starvation, provoked an outcry.

I was convinced that nutrition should be taken out of politics and that this could be done by an accurate knowledge of the facts. As we had not got the facts, in 1946 I decided to carry out a National Nutritional Survey. I submitted a project to the ministerial authorities and they approved. The survey was entrusted to Dr Desmond Hourihane of the Department. To ensure that there could be no criticism because of bias or anything else we brought the Medical Research Council into it and they set up an advisory committee. Dr Hourihane put a tremendous amount of work into this project and for a few years this was his life. To my mind it was one of the best nutritional surveys ever carried out anywhere.

We received magnificent help and cooperation from the British Ministry of Health who were interested to see whether their survey methods would work in another country. But I believe that Des Hourihane improved on even their high standards. Mathematical sampling had not long begun and Roy Geary and the Central Statistics Office had rapidly become very expert in this field. They were able to give for the whole country, on a balanced sample basis, an exact selection of households to be examined for their food consumption. They also machined and carried out any mathematical analysis Des Hourihane needed.

This survey put us in possession of the facts on the food patterns of the Irish, the deficiencies, where they existed and the people who were affected. It showed that, in contrast to the rest of Europe, the Irish were very well fed indeed. We had no idea that things were as good as they were. It was borne out many years later by the World Health Organisation who showed that it was a toss-up whether it was the Australians or the Irish who were the best-fed people in the world.

On the other hand, we had large families of children, of unemployed or poorly paid people, who did not have enough. The problem of rickets in Dublin was confirmed and explained by the shortage of calcium in the diet of such people. However, relative to the over-all situation, these problems were minor. They also affected some old people, not because they could not buy food, but because they were old, living alone and had no effective cooking facilities. The main thing was to care for the children in large families.

4

National Health Planning — Irish Style

Early in 1945 Dr Ward and Mr MacEntee asked me to prepare a plan for the development of the National Health Services. This was part of a general effort for the post-war development of the country. Each Department was asked to prepare a development plan for the field with which it was concerned.

I was too green and inexperienced to undertake this myself and asked for help. In the event a committee was set up which included John Collins who afterwards became Secretary of the Department of Local Government and Public Health, P.J. Keady who was later Secretary of the Department of Social Welfare, John Garvin who also became Secretary of the Department, and myself. A fairly formidable lot. We had Des Roche as secretary of the group. We held seventeen full meetings and eleven meetings of a sub-committee and produced a report in September 1945. One of the interesting things we found when we examined the health services of advanced countries was that there had been an unprecedented movement in this field all over the world. Commencing with the New Zealand Social Security Act of 1938 to provide for a complete Social Security and Health Service, on to the British White Paper 'A National Health Service' of 1944 most of the advanced countries had attempted some kind of development. Sir William Beveridge's report of 1942, 'Social Insurance and Allied Services', which advocated a health service to which people would have access on the basis of need rather than ability to pay, had a profound influence on the English-speaking world.

It is interesting to reflect on why this should have occurred. Perhaps it was due to an excess of sickness after the depression and during and after the Second World War. In those circumstances people began to discover the striking mismatch between the potential of medical science to improve health and the actuality, full of inefficiencies and inequities. Governments gradually became more socially concerned. Advances in organisation and administration made it possible to provide public health schemes and medical care coverage. Countries with health schemes already tried to improve them and to bring them up to date. This was not a matter of ideology since right-wing countries like Spain were as interested as socialist countries like the USSR.

There were two broad methods of financing these new health schemes. One was the insurance method, most popular in Western European countries, but which had never really developed in this country as a means of funding health services. The other, a universally available service financed out of central or local taxation. The latter was adopted by New Zealand and the UK. Canada adopted a scheme with elements of both methods.

Shortly before we began work there had been two developments. In October 1944 the Medical Association of Ireland submitted to the Minister a scheme for an improved health service. In early 1945 Dr John Dignan, the Bishop of Clonfert and Chairman of the National Health Insurance Society, also sent Mr MacEntee (with a good deal of publicity) a comprehensive plan for Social Insurance, which included a radical change in the nation's health services.

Dr Dignan's Social Security Scheme largely followed the continental pattern of national insurance. He proposed a National Insurance Corporation to administer all social services including the health services. It was in effect a welfare state to cover everyone who was employed, from 16 to 65, and their dependants. It was to be compulsory. Those who were self-employed could become voluntary contributors. In effect it was to be a vast expansion of the National Health Insurance Society, which had been established some years before to provide for the amalgamation of the very large number of small voluntary or friendly or commerical insurance bodies, which had provided different social and health coverage for insured workers. Despite its name, the range of health benefits provided through the National Health Insurance Society was extremely limited.

Dr Dignan proposed that there should be a Minister for

the Social Services, a Central Insurance Board as well as the
Corporation, but the relationship between the three was not
well worked out. From the political point of view, it really
removed all health and welfare from the Minister's control
and vested it in the new Board and its operating body, the
Corporation, and this the political authorities were not prepared to accept. Anyway, it was clear that the existing
National Health Insurance Society neither had sufficient
experience nor was their organisation, even if expanded,
capable of undertaking the running of the social and health
services of the country. Mr MacEntee considered that the
Bishop had not been asked to prepare any such scheme and
had exceeded his mandate as chairman of the Society. In any
case he was annoyed to have this thing sprung on him. When
the chairmanship of the National Health Insurance Society
next became vacant, Dr Dignan was not reappointed.

The plan or scheme of the Medical Association of Ireland
could have been drawn up at the Clongowes Social Order
Summer School. It proposed a Ministry of Health with a
Minister, a Central Health Council, a Medical Chief Executive and four Assistant Medical Commissioners. It stated
that the main reason for establishing the Council was to
ensure a vocational as opposed to what was called a bureaucratic organisation of the health services. It was a purely
'corporate' approach and the only place where I found this
philosophy in my travels was in Eastern Europe, particularly
the USSR. The scheme proposed a general practitioner service
which combined the dispensary service with insurance cover
for those on moderate incomes, with doctors paid a mixture of
salary and capitation payments.

There were many good points in the Association's Scheme
but the main object of it was to place the medical profession
solidly in charge of the health services. Many people all over
the world would regard this as making sense but it was certainly
not acceptable to the political authorities or the administrators
here. One fundamental problem which the Scheme did not
address was how to ensure access to hospital and specialist
services by those on moderate incomes for whom hospital
and medical bills could be crippling financially.

Our committee more or less wrote its own terms of reference

which were: 1. To study the existing medical services; 2. To study trends in developments in other countries; 3. To study schemes of improvement submitted by non-official bodies (the Bishop's and the Medical Association's); 4. To make official proposals, 5. To review the financial and administrative measures necessary to give effect to the official recommendations.

In considering a reorganisation of the health services in any country, there are several factors to be considered. The first is, that there already exists a cadre of medical personnel, trained to carry out their functions and that you are stuck with them. You cannot take them out and shoot them, therefore you have to work with what you have and must make the best use you can of this force. It is useless for Ministers of Health, as is their custom all over the world, to try to advance their own political creed, or to court popularity, by bullying or doctor-bashing. The vast majority of doctors are hard-working men and women, normal, decent people and are really concerned for their patients. The world over, doctors do try to make a go of even the daftest ideas of Ministers of Health and the administrators in their Departments. I include in this nurses and all the range of professional and technical personnel working in the health field. After a life-time of experience working all over the world, I am as convinced today as I was forty years ago that the only way to make progress is to give due recognition to the views of the professional people concerned in a service and to ensure their participation in developing it. It is essential to ensure that they receive equitable and fair treatment in determining purposes and goals.

Secondly, health services generally lack a statement or definition of what they hope to achieve, beyond vague aspirations as to improving or providing good health. Doctors simply go on doing their old job in their old way, the way they were trained and that's that. We wanted to express the public health aims of the service in as clear a way as possible.

Thirdly, we felt the need for a national health plan to prevent local, political, professional and institutional influences skewing our efforts. When I came into the Department I found that people had been thinking about the health services since the beginning of the state. The Hospitals Commission had issued two excellent reports on *Hospital Planning*. My predecessors had made wise recommendations in the Department, sometimes they were followed and when they were not we were stuck with the consequences.

A fourth objective was that an attempt should be made to correct the fragmentation of the health services. We had more or less separate public health services, a dispensary service, private practitioners, medical schools, research, voluntary hospitals, public assistance institutions, a range of specialist institutions and specialists, such as tuberculosis, infectious diseases and orthopaedic, and the mental hospitals were a separate preserve governed by their own legal statutes. Lastly there was the national health insurance, which provided certain health benefits for insured persons. These schemes were more often than not under different managements and had insufficient common purpose or interest.

A fifth consideration was that the existing medical services were largely curative and their preventive aspects were not sufficiently developed. Greater efforts were needed to promote the health of the individual and of the community. I felt that the social implications of medicine should be more appreciated and that greater achievement in detecting and arresting disease at the first onset was now possible. The family doctor of the future should I believed, in addition to an interest in the mental, social and physical well-being of the community, by taking routine examination of all patients, say once a year, endeavour to detect degenerative disease in its early treatable stages. By ante-natal examinations, immunisation, the regular examination and treatment of defects in pre-school and school children and by a general programme of health promotion, the doctor would influence community health to a greater extent than by the treatment of disease amongst already sick people. Later, a mass-radiography and the prevention of heart disease and hypertension by health education and regular checks as well as ante-natal care showed how this might have worked.

Sixthly, we wanted the services of medical specialists to be more readily available to the ordinary public. In 1945, specialist services were grossly inadequate throughout the country and were not readily available to the ordinary patient. Outside of

Dublin they barely existed. Both practitioner and specialist are required: the one for early diagnosis and a proportion of the treatment, for after-care and the treatment of disease in its family and community setting, the other for specialist care in the hospital situation.

On the other hand, the ideal of the family doctor was to be preserved and encouraged. I considered that the medical services based on the family doctor should be locally administered, not controlled by a remote centralised bureaucracy. The strong personal element characteristic of Irish medicine, as it was in 1945, was shown by the attachment of the people to their doctors. Local medical men and women possess enormous power to do good by reason of this faith and it is essential to preserve and utilise this personal relationship. The family doctor cannot be superseded by any other agency, at least so far as Ireland is concerned.

Finally, it was advocated that hospital and specialist services should be administered on a regional basis. In 1945, they were organised on a county or county borough system and were handicapped by this arrangement.

In our proposals, it was recommended that a number of general practitioner units should be established in each county. Each unit should be related to the community and consist of say 700 households and that for each a medical officer, a district nurse and a midwife should be available. My colleagues and I outlined the duties of the District Medical Officer/Family Doctor. In addition to treating sickness amongst his patients he or she would provide a wide range of services: ante-natal and maternity; welfare care of infants and children under school age; periodic inspection and treatment of school children; immunisation of children; annual medical survey of the members of each family; investigation of matters affecting health and vital statistics in the district and reporting on these to the County Medical Officer; being familiar with the family circumstances, habits, heredity and disease reactions in the district; assisting in the case-finding of tuberculosis and other diseases and being concerned with the source and control of infection in the area; assisting in education for the promotion and maintenance of health; correlating and assisting in the administration of the various social services insofar as they

concerned the public health; superintending the work of the
district nurse and midwife; medical certification for national
health insurance and other purposes. We proposed that there
should be group practices, where possible from clinics, freedom of choice of doctor, the right to private practice by
doctors, help from assistant medical officers and so on.

Another thing I wanted was that there should be a post-
graduate medical centre, where practitioners could come for
resident refresher courses in St James' Hospital, because of
the wonderful clinical material there. They would learn new
techniques in treatment, minor surgery and anything new
which might add to their ability to serve their patients. This
was to ensure that all practitioners would be kept up-to-date
and would not have to rely exclusively for their post-graduate
instruction on the representatives of the pharmaceutical companies. It was not proposed that this amenity would in any
way be under the direction of the Department.

The main idea was that the general practitioner would be
responsible for the health of the individual, the family and
the community. In addition to duties in curing disease, the
doctor would have a positive role in prevention.

One inspiration for the concept was the work and life of
men like Dr Sam Agnew of Lurgan. Sometime after the passing
of the 1878 Health Act, Agnew made the town landlords
clean up their properties. They had to tear down every second
back-to-back house, to provide water supplies and water
closets and yards. He changed the lives of the poor people of
Lurgan. He was a general practitioner and he was a dispensary
doctor but he was also the Medical Officer of Health for the
town. In a time of poverty and hunger, scarletina, diphtheria,
rampant TB and terrible infant mortality, a time of shocking
housing conditions, tramps, filthy lodging houses and open
sewers running down into the Lough, he had the courage to
clean up the town. Sam Agnew, whom my father loved, is
forgotten, but he was a truly great man.

The administrative and financial aspects of the report were
largely the work of my colleagues. Influenced by current thinking we looked forward to the entire population being covered
gradually by a service without charge, as in New Zealand, the
UK and elsewhere. The development was to be approached

in stages and was to be, as in Canada, partly financed by insurance contributions and partly by state funds both central and local. It was particularly tailored for Irish society and was a neat and economical job. We proposed to provide hospitals at four levels, regional, secondary in large centres, and county and district. For the first two we would have a comprehensive specialist staffing. Each county hospital would have a specialist surgeon, physician and obstetrician. They would not engage in general practice and would see only cases referred to them by general practitioners. The regional hospitals in Cork and Galway would be related to medical teaching centres, so that the Professors of Medicine and Surgery would be the seniors in the regional hierarchy and the Professor of Paediatrics, for instance, would be the senior paediatrician in the regional paediatric specialist service and so on. We had as aspirations the creation of effective specialist services, the integration of these services with the medical schools and the complete coverage of the population as regards class, geography or whatever.

The Report was submitted in December 1945 in something of a hurry because the Government wanted to see it. Its publication met with opposition in Cabinet. None of us was told very much about why, except that it was unacceptable, and with the hint that the Minister of Finance opposed it. It seems strange now that the product of the hard work, over months, of four or five of the most senior civil servants in the country, on a vital matter for the future well-being of the national community, could be dismissed without explanation, discussion or any kind of hearing. It also seems wrong that there was no discussion with the Medical Association about their scheme. As for the poor Bishop, there was something of an outcry about the highhanded way in which he was treated by Mr. MacEntee. As an alternative to our Report, I was asked to submit proposals for reforming the health services in the form of a draft White Paper. The issues we had raised clearly influenced Mr. De Valera. In January 1946 he announced that a new and separate Department of Health would be established. Our Report would provide the rationale for that Department. Our proposals, in a modified form were published in the White Paper, *Outline of Proposals for the Improvement of the Health*

Services, published in 1947 and were given a statutory basis in the Health Acts, 1947 and 1952 and the Health (Financial Provisions) Act, 1947.

In the meantime I quietly went ahead and began implementing our proposals anyway, with the encouragement of the Minister. The problems were there and I just could not look at them and do nothing. The patient needed treatment and the patient got it. So apart from the general practitioner reform, the rest was carried out. We built the hospitals according to the programme, and gradually created the specialist service as we outlined. We developed the specialist service on a regional basis so that when it was functioning it became necessary to create a regional system of administration. The money from the Sweep, which was under the effective control of the Minister gave us a measure of independence from the Department of Finance's veto. Although it was turned down by the Cabinet in 1945, the service today is very much as we planned it then. Under a succession of different Ministers we quietly went ahead and organised it this way. Nobody said anything, and we just did it and they all seemed to approve. Tom Barrington, who watched all this over the years, called it 'National Health Planning — Irish Style'.

The only failure in the plan and one which I bitterly regretted was the follow-up of the preventive side of the general practitioner service and indeed of the reorganisation of this aspect of medicine. Our dispensary service had been unaltered for more than a hundred years. There were between 800 and 1,000 doctors in this service. One third were 70 years of age or more. Owing to the war, a third of the dispensaries had only temporary medical officers serving and the remaining third were in such a frame of mind that a decent scheme would not have been opposed and the Medical Association welcomed a change. So there was an unusual opportunity to make a change.

The medical needs of the people were changing and because of population shifts the siting of dispensaries or clinics needed review. We needed to know more about the operation of group practice and the views of the doctors were necessary and how, from their own experience, did they think that things could be improved? This was a wonderful opportunity to revolutionise the general practice care of the population, but we needed facts and ideas as well as the cooperation of the doctors in effecting change. We would in the course of this exercise have had a reasonable hope of interesting them in the Mother and Child Scheme and in the concept of community care, a thing that was never done properly.

What I really wanted to do was to come up with a model which would enable us to make a steady, regular improvement in personal and community health. It had been my criticism of various national health services that they were not really organised to do this. Medicine went on largely as before except that it became free for most people, but it did not produce any marked results in improving health and was often bad value for money.

In the early days of the Department of Health, about the end of 1947 when we had recruited the additional medical inspectors, I started a dispensary survey. Each of the medical inspectors of the Department studied the counties for which he was responsible. In discussion with the local doctors they sought to find the trends of medical problems in the different districts, the needs of the people, the omissions, the successes and the failures. We studied also the population and community changes in areas, as well as geographical and social and economic developments in an attempt to map out the new health bailiwicks. When we had finished the country areas, we intended to study Dublin, Cork and other places. We got about half-way through examining the counties, the material was coming in and things were beginning to take shape when relations within the Department became somewhat difficult and I was invited to leave and to take up duties outside. When I left, for one reason or another the survey ended. It seems a pity now because had we been able to finish it there is no doubt that we would have come up with facts and ideas on which we would have been able to make proposals.

In implementing the other parts of the plan we began with the specialist services and the staffing of the county hospitals. These posts were filled, sometimes by the retirement or superannuation of the existing holders of posts and by their replacement, sometimes by the creation of new posts or sometimes by the building of new hospitals and the need to staff them.

In the dispensary service it became necessary to fill posts and we raised the standards by looking for doctors with longer and more varied experience and training. Through the Local Appointments Commission we specified that general practitioner applicants should have special experience or training in child health, tuberculosis and/or public health. The posts were awarded on merit and so great became the competition that people went off and got the special training or sat for the particular qualification needed. After some years we had a really superbly trained, experienced and qualified cadre of physicians, surgeons and other specialists in different fields. Our staff of practitioners could hold their own with the finest anywhere. It was they who made our health service one of the best in the world. When you provide new hospitals and equipment and staff the operation with first-class men and women and put them to work in the right atmosphere of things being done and things happening, then you can't lose.

There were many things responsible for this happy situation. One was that there had been a series of enlightened Ministers in the Custom House, they had introduced really good legislation which set up for example the Local Appointments Commission and the Civil Service Commissions which had had a splendid effect in that appointments were made on merit. They had welcomed the Rockefeller aid and had built up a splendid team of public health people. They fought through various Health Acts and displayed a lot of courage in doing so. They were hard workers themselves and wise men, even though at times they were too quarrelsome and apt to take offence, nevertheless they did a good job. Equally there were highly experienced, skilled and honest, intelligent administrators and the relations with the technocrats were good. Anyway, the whole set-up was sensible, and if imperfect, was made to work and worked well.

The Maternity Care Scheme
When our plan for a National Health Service had been rejected by the Cabinet Dr Ward asked me to try again and aim for something more modest. This was in October 1945. By this time I had more knowledge of the situation, of the needs and the priorities.

In Ireland at that time relative to the population we had one of the lowest marriage rates in the world. When people did marry, they married relatively late in life. Then we had one of the highest birth rates per family. These basic demographic factors created a whole host of problems. It meant that from the total population a small number of parents had the burden of rearing the vast bulk of the future generation. There were a large number of older women rearing large families and at risk because of late pregnancies. People with large families were almost always, of necessity, poor and because of this poverty many children suffered.

There were other factors. The women who were able to attend the three lying-in hospitals in Dublin received excellent ante-natal care if they came for it, but with the vast majority of births in the country care was inadequate and in consequence too many women died in childbirth. One-third of all beds in the three lying-in hospitals in Dublin at that time were occupied by 'waiting cases', women who had toxaemia of pregnancy, malnutrition, anaemia or a host of other things where it was necessary to bring them into hospital for a few weeks and to treat them to build up their health before their deliveries. Lack of ante-natal care or an inadequate attention meant that the health of such women could become permanently impaired.

In those days no one even thought of the concept of peri-natal mortality and the infant mortality rate and particularly the mortality of infants in the first month of life was far too high. As the Belfast Infant Mortality Study had shown, even at that time 70 per cent of babies could have been saved. Care of infants in hospital, apart from the two or three specialist children's hospitals, was quite inadequate. In Dublin every year 600 babies died from enteritis alone. As a consequence of the lack of ante-natal care and the generally poor mid-wifery and the state of health of the poorer women, due to war-time privation, many required repair operations which for one reason or another they did not receive.

The Schools Medical Services examinations of children showed that as many as 8,000 children each year showed heart defects and another group of the same size had chest diseases, either chronic bronchitis, asthma or other such conditions. In addition to these two groups there were a great number of children who were generally unhealthy. The vast majority of all these conditions, many of which would handicap a child for life, began in the pre-school or 'toddler' age and could have been prevented. The Belfast Survey had confirmed that it was the children of the poor, of large families living in poor areas, who died.

From a study of the Dublin Corporation Maternity and Child Welfare Centres, which I made at the time, I found that only about 20 per cent of those for whom they were intended used the centres. The Belfast experience had shown the importance of nursing for infants who were sick and at risk and of the necessity of surveillance, since the clinical condition of a child could change so dramatically in such a short time. The Dublin Nursing Service was, to say the least, quite inadequate. There were plenty of nurses available but the operation was badly organised. Finally, the North of Ireland experience had shown that when the free medical care scheme was introduced for insured workers, the so-called panel system, it was really the wives and children who needed the service. Certainly, in times of stress they needed it, far more than the insured workers. Despite this the free service was confined to employed or unemployed workers.

This was the situation which brought me to recommend, as a priority, a White Paper describing a scheme for the care of women and children and which I produced in the spring of 1946. The main object was to ensure a healthy rising generation and to repair the damage which the hardship of war-time conditions had caused to the vulnerable groups of women and children. One day I was walking up to Bewley's for a coffee and a bun lunch and as usual I was accompanied by J.D. MacCormack. I had been working all morning on the White Paper and it was very much on my mind. As I passed Maxwell Weldon's the solicitors on Eden Quay, I said to J.D. quite suddenly, 'I've got to name this thing. We'll call it the Mother and Child Service; that should sell it, no one could oppose a scheme with a name like that.'

Under the scheme the Government would provide a free comprehensive obstetric service of ante-natal, delivery and post-natal care for every woman. Child care would be based on proper home visiting of infants failing to thrive, surveillance of pre-school children and provision of medical care for any defects found, proper immunisation against preventable diseases, regular examination of school children and treatment for any defects found. All this and anything else that I could think of, including free medical care for all youngsters up to the age of sixteen years, was in the scheme. The whole was to be provided in a well-organised national service, making sure that every woman and child was covered free, in a thorough manner. The White Paper was published in 1947.

On my return from America in the autumn of 1946 we started to implement the scheme. The first thing I did was to recommend to Dr Ward that the three lying-in hospitals of the City of Dublin, which cared for 80 per cent of all births in the city should inaugurate a new infant service. The idea was, as the Belfast Survey had shown, that it should be possible to identify the infants at risk from key factors such as low birth weights, difficult births, history of previous infant deaths in the family and so on. Infants failing to gain weight should not be allowed to remain at home under the unskilled care of a young mother but should receive expert nursing in a special infant unit until they were going along well. In the meantime the mother would receive some training in child care. I recommended that the hospitals should take over the care of the infants for the first month and that a staff be trained and employed to carry out regular home visiting, paying particular attention to those children at risk. Each hospital should have a small intensive care unit, separate from the hospital, so that any infection going should not be brought in from outside. The unit would be staffed with specially trained nurses and equipped with sufficient incubators to look after babies who were found not to be thriving. Children were at the maximum risk during the first month of birth and particularly the first week, and so it was necessary to provide for a continuity of care.

Dr Ward liked the idea, (as did Mr MacEntee) and the Masters of the three hospitals were invited to meet him in the Dáil one evening late in his office. Ninian Faulkner of the Rotunda, Alec Spain of the National Maternity in Holles Street and Eddie Keelan, the Master of the Coombe, attended. We had a great session, they were enthusiastic and the whole thing was planned there and then. The three Masters sold the idea to their Boards of Governors and by 1947 most of it was in operation and working. It certainly saved a great number of lives. This was done by the hard work and expert care which the staffs of the three hospitals gave to these sick scraps of humanity, often fighting desperately for their lives. It was heartening to go into one of these units and see a dozen or so babies doing well in incubators and know that a few months before they would have died.

We started training schemes in neonatal care and brought up nursing staffs from all over the country to take part in these exercises. We added equipment like incubators anywhere they were needed and generally began a drive to save infant lives. From what I had seen during my Rockefeller trip in the Johns Hopkins Hospital in Baltimore with Professor Parks and his cubicles for sick infants and barrier nursing I tried to popularise this too, and in any new hospitals I personally designed the infants' units as well as trying to put them into older hospitals where I could.

I visited various medical societies in places like Cork and Galway to explain what it was all about. All this bore fruit in all kinds of ways. Bob Collis wrote a training manual *Neonatal Care for Nurses*, the paediatricians and the Masters became interested and advanced the cause and their contributions and ideas moved things on. The Archbishop of Dublin, Dr John Charles McQuaid, regarded with a certain amount of suspicion by the liberal element amongst the medicals, sponsored the building of a magnificent Children's Hospital at Crumlin in Dublin. However when they had finished it they had too many children's beds and not enough cots and we had to help reorganise it to meet proper needs of the disease situation as it was then.

We extended, as a first phase in our scheme, maternity accommodation in district and other institutions to provide for a minimum of 50 per cent of all births. Forty years ago that was an enlightened provision by any standard anywhere.

Health Education
One of the issues in child care that concerned me was health

education. There was no use teaching boys and girls to read and write if at the same time you did not teach them hygiene and the adoption of simple healthy habits. When on the Rockefeller Foundation Fellowship I found that in Boston, New York, Baltimore and Philadelphia the school authorities of the catholic schools, the public health people and the teachers had all come together to produce health education courses. These were contained in manuals supplied to all teachers and in the schools the teaching was used to pass on the health instruction. In addition to having the imprint of the health and educational people they had the ecclesiastical imprimatur. I found these books very good and brought copies home with me. They did however relate to the American scene.

To start the teaching of health to Irish children we decided to draw up courses more in keeping with our own traditions and needs. To do this we decided to hold, for a beginning, a Summer School for Deans of boys' boarding schools the following year. I visited Clongowes, Castleknock and Blackrock and saw the heads of these schools and they agreed to participate. I then visited Canon Ryan of St Kieran's in Kilkenny, the Chairman of the Standing Committee of the Catholic Headmasters. He gave the idea enthusiastic support, especially when he saw my American books on the subject with the imprimaturs of Cardinals and Archbishops across the Atlantic.

We were going to hold the first Summer School in Blackrock College and representatives would be invited from all the boys' boarding schools in the country. This was to be the first step. Next year we would do the girls' boarding schools and so on, gradually working our way to the primary grade. The reception at the start was encouraging and all was set to go ahead when John Garvin pointed out that we had no budget to finance such an enterprise. Neither had we legal powers. So he drafted a section to be included in the Health Bill of 1947. The section gave a legal basis for a nation-wide mother and child health service and for educating mothers and children about health. The Bill obliged health authorities to 'make arrangements for safe-guarding the health of women in respect of motherhood and for their education in that respect' and to provide a comprehensive health and health-education service for children before and during their school years. This was the section of the Bill which provoked such controversy. As the Bill was concerned with the establishment of a Mother and Child Scheme we had to relate the section on health education to education in respect of maternal and child health, which possibly gave it an ambiguous meaning. In 1947 the Catholic Hierarchy condemned this section as posing a danger to the morals of women and children. They feared that it would open the door to information on contraception and abortion. The origin of the section dealing with Health Education in the Health Act of 1947, shows that, initially the clergy were not against health education, until the medical politicians inspired their opposition.

Nursing Developments

I was convinced that an effective nursing service was essential for the care of infants and to enable us to reduce the deaths. In Ireland nursing training was very good indeed and was in the hands of the major hospitals. Indeed, Florence Nightingale did her training here with the Irish Sisters of Charity. The body which 'headed-up' the nursing profession was largely medically controlled and was merely an examining and qualifying Board. It had little or no control over the hospital training schools and the standard could vary from places like St Vincent's, equal to the best in the world, to other places of less quality.

The only funds the Board had were the fees collected for examining and qualifying the nurses and registering them. The midwives had a separate body and were controlled by the Central Midwives Board, again largely consisting of medical people. They set the standards, defined the rules, penalised midwives reported to them for infringements of the rules, and carried out examinations. This Board had played a great part in moving midwifery from the untrained 'handywoman' up to the well-trained, technically qualified birth-attendant. However it had become an anachronism.

When Queen Victoria achieved her Diamond Jubilee the women of Ireland gave her a large sum of money as a present. This she handed back, as she was not short of cash at the time and with great foresight said that she would like to see it spent on the creation of a district nursing service, particularly for the sick poor. In this way the Jubilee Nursing Service was created and it is fair to testify to the wonderful work of this organisation over the years. It included several hundred district nurses. They had their own training school, had a high standard of work, were extraordinarily dedicated and were beloved by the people they served. A smaller service, equally good, existed in districts in the west, founded by Lady Dudley, wife of one of the viceroys.

In addition to these two organisations there were two others. One consisted of the public health nurses, working with the county medical officers of health and dealing with school inspections and hygiene, tuberculosis and infectious diseases. Dublin Corporation had its own large but relatively inefficient district nursing service.

The problem was that the funds of the Jubilee and the Dudley organisations were drying up and, as there was an element of former ascendancy 'patronage' in their management, the politicians were not too keen on them. In any case it was necessary to graft a larger content of public health, hygiene and disease prevention on to their work. Equally it was necessary to influence the public health nurses with the dedication and devotion of the Jubilees, so that they would not become mere local officials, bureaucrats rather than good and real nurses.

So I worked out a scheme to combine the whole thing into an organised, nation-wide nursing service. It was proposed to set up a Central Nursing Authority to be controlled by the nurses themselves. This would have the power to control nursing standards, training and development and it would have the necessary funds. This scheme was turned into an excellent Bill by Tom Brady and was piloted through the Dáil by Dr James Ryan the then Minister of Health. The Act enabled us to set up An Bord Altranais, the National Nursing Board. In a short time we had a service of District Public Health Nurses combining public health work with the excellent domiciliary care hitherto given by the Jubilees. We also managed the appointment of a Nursing Officer in the Department, Miss Reidy. All this took a bit of organising and J.D. MacCormack, Des Hourihane and Harry O'Flanagan and of course later, Miss Reidy, were very busy setting it up with the County Health

Officers. The passing of the Act and the appointment of Miss Reidy were a very great advance for the nursing profession.

The Irish Nurses Organisation decided to welcome Miss Reidy with a formal luncheon and arranged that afterwards there would be a mass meeting of nurses which I should address. I was to tell them the good news of their enhanced professional status. The lunch was held, speeches were made welcoming Miss Reidy and so on by the leaders of the nursing profession, particularly by Miss Nelly Healy, a wonderful lady, and then we made our way to the meeting. Peg Reidy clutched a bouquet of flowers almost as big as herself and which I remember consisted largely of 'Love-in-the-mist', which I thought at the time was highly appropriate. The mass meeting turned out to consist of seven nurses. To further show their appreciation of the whole thing, at the first election of the new Bord Altranais they returned the same old matrons and the same old medical faces.

We were so full of the idea of nursing services playing an important role in the future health services of the world that, at the second assembly of the World Health Organisation in 1950, Dr J.D. MacCormack of the Irish Delegation proposed that nurses should be appointed to the staff of WHO. He got it carried by judicious lobbying, at which J.D. was unsurpassed. This was something wonderful since up to that, throughout much of the world, nurses had been regarded as uneducated hospital servants and in Muslim countries they had a very bad reputation indeed.

Later I took every opportunity when addressing matron groups and people like that to harangue them on their responsibility, not only to train the young women (there were no male nurses then) in their charge as nurses, but also to educate them. If a girl could sing or perhaps play the violin she should be encouraged to do some musical studies. They should be taken to such places as the National Gallery, taught civics, taken to the Dáil to see how the country is governed and so on. On graduation they should be well-educated and informed people. Later, if they married and settled down, say in a rural area, they would become valuable community leaders. It was important that they should see that student nurses were not exploited as cheap labour. I used to watch the old battle-axes of matrons as I expounded these doctrines and see a glazed look come over their eyes as they stifled the odd yawn. They would look at one another and I could imagine them saying 'here he goes again'.

5

The Campaign Against Tuberculosis Begins

The existence of a tuberculosis problem in Ireland had been recognised since 1841 when the first Census indicated that 14,000 deaths each year were due to the disease, out of a population of eight millions. As the population fell due to famine and emigration, deaths were reduced to 10,000 in 1861. Until the end of the nineteenth century no special provision was made for tuberculosis and cases were either treated at home by general practitioners or dispensary doctors, or in workhouse hospitals, charitable institutions and general hospitals. The Public Health Act of 1878 did not list tuberculosis as a 'notifiable disease'.

After Koch's discovery of the tubercle bacillus in 1882 there was a world-wide awakening of interest in the disease. In Ireland, following on a public meeting in the College of Physicians, the first sanatorium was established at Newcastle, County Wicklow, in 1896. There were international congresses in London (1901) and Paris (1908) and Ireland was represented. The Cork City and County authorities combined to set up Heatherside Sanatorium at Doneraile in 1904 and Dublin City and County established Crooksling Sanatorium in 1907. The Pigeon House Sanatorium was opened in 1907 and was built on the benefaction of Allan A. Ryan of New York.

Lady Aberdeen, wife of the Viceroy, became interested in tuberculosis and helped to set up the Women's National Health Association. My mother was involved as secretary of the Lurgan Branch. This body organised a Tuberculosis Exhibition in Dublin in 1907 as part of the International Exhibition held at that time. Later the tuberculosis section of the exhibition travelled to all the main towns of Ireland. On the suggestion of the Gaelic League Dr O'Beirne of Leenane was appointed to travel all over the Gaeltacht to lecture in Irish on tuberculosis. The hardships he endured there brought about his early death.

The Women's National Health Association provided the stimulus to build Peamount Sanatorium in Newcastle, Co Dublin, in 1912 and funded an industrial establishment set up for the training of patients for industry in that institution. The work of the Association became world-famous when at the Tuberculosis Conference in Washington in 1908 they shared the Grand Prize for voluntary work with the TB Association of New York.

As the result of the increase in tuberculosis from a rate of 165 per 100,000 of the population to 277 per 100,000 at the end of the century, pressure from the Women's National Health Association and agitation by the medical profession, leading to deputations to the Viceroy and other activities, the Tuberculosis Prevention Act (Ireland) was passed in 1908. This was a simple Act authorising County Councils to provide sanatoria, hospitals, dispensaries and to employ staff, to provide bacteriological services, veterinary services to control meat and milk, to provide drugs and to conduct education in preventing tuberculosis. It did not include compulsory notification of cases. It could be accepted or rejected by a County Council. No money was made available apart from a possible rate of a penny in the pound valuation. Voluntary notification did not work. As Des Roche wrote on this period, 'The onus of educating people regarding the disease was thrown on the sanitary authorities, a legislative instance of the blind being requested to lead the blind'. There was no central directing authority (although one was sought by Professor MacWeeney) and in effect things happened slowly. There was no specific treatment available and the emphasis was on fresh air, bed rest, hygiene and sojourn in the mountains, preferably amongst pine trees.

The first phase of the development of the Irish tuberculosis services marked the participation of Ireland in a growing international awareness of tuberculosis. The movement was an enlightened and compassionate awakening of the middle classes, hitherto little responsive to the sufferings of the vast multitude of the poor in Ireland. The movement had political overtones in that it happened during a Liberal administration in the UK and it was a safe thing about which to agitate. It had the blessing of the vice reine and there was always the prospect of the odd knighthood in the offing. Theo MacWeeney's father, a tremendous figure in the movement, was never so rewarded. I think he talked too much sense and was too much of a maverick to receive favours. But it was a distinguishable national social effort by people who had never lifted a finger to help anyone before, at least in tuberculosis. It was enlightened in that it tried to get away from the Poor Law and entrusted the care of tuberculosis to the County Councils.

By 1911 a synthesis began to emerge with the passing of the National Health Insurance Act, which provided sanatorium benefit for insured persons, set up committees to administer the Act and for the first time put up some money for the County Councils. Thereafter, bit by bit, councils appointed whole-time tuberculosis officers, opened small sanatoria or participated in the opening or maintenance of places like Peamount, provided laboratory services, food supplements and tuberculosis dispensaries. Each year in one way or another they received help to keep the service going.

The service worked well according to the standards of those days, and the death rate fell from 277 in 1900 to 165 per 100,000 of the population in 1920, though conditions were patchy. I can remember as a boy Drs Robinson and Gillespie, tuberculosis officers for the counties of Armagh and Down respectively, calling with my father to discuss cases and their interest and the exemplary care they showed for patients. Dr Gillespie was a great advocate of tuberculin treatment, something long forgotten. When later I went into practice I became a member of the Co Armagh Tuberculosis Committee, a singularly ineffective body.

When the Free State was established the Rockefeller Foundation supported the beginning of a county health service in 1926. Four public health officers were sent to America to train, one of them being Austin Harbinson, later a very good friend of mine. When these men came back from Harvard or Yale they set such an example that soon the whole country was covered by an excellent public health service.

Each county had a CMO and usually an assistant CMO with several public health nurses. These people took over the tuberculosis service, ran the local sanatoria and provided domiciliary care. Until the coming of the Second World War the death rate declined steadily. According to the ideas and social standards of the times people were reasonably cared for. The Irish service, if a bit homespun, was as good as if not better than the services existing in other countries which could be compared with Ireland.

During the Second World War, as in the First, there was a marked increase in the morbidity and mortality from the disease. Faced with this increase and the difficult war-time conditions the service was quite unable to cope. We had an influx of Irish people returning from abroad suffering from the disease which made things worse. Between 1942 and 1945, 16,186 people died of the disease. It was clear that something should be done.

In 1942 the Royal Academy of Medicine presented to the Minister of Local Government and Public Health a scheme for the detection, cure and prevention of tuberculosis. Again in December 1943 the anti-tuberculosis section of the Irish Red Cross Society presented a report containing the outlines of a long-term tuberculosis scheme. The Hospitals Commission in their second report submitted a scheme comprising the building of regional sanatoria, a central chest hospital, chest hospital units and improved local sanatoria for chronic and advanced cases at a rate of providing one bed per annual death.

In 1944 there were approximately 3,000 TB beds in 52 institutions, mainly small local sanatoria. During the war the condition of these small sanatoria had deteriorated and as regards the care of patients the situation was downright bad.

To visit some of these places and to see long lines of people, mainly young men and women, in bed in the old-fashioned wards, under miserable conditions, without even a hot-water bottle in winter, hopeless and helpless, most of them slowly dying, was heart-breaking. In the odd place, particularly where the staff were not defeated, were kindly and caring, things were better, but generally institutions were feared as 'death-houses'. Few came out alive. There was great frustration among the medical people and everyone you met had his or her 'hang-up' with the system.

As Chief Medical Adviser to the Department I found myself

in the midst of a situation of conflicting reports, proposals and pressure groups. In addition there was mounting public indignation. The government had been holding on, hoping that the problem would go away and then considering 'kicking for touch' by handing the whole thing over to the Irish Red Cross and thus washing their hands of it. It was apparent to me however that such a problem could not be handled by any purely voluntary body, without an organisation, staff or knowledge. TB was far too serious an issue to play games with. It had to be faced.

Early in 1945 when I had a chance to look the thing over with help from Theo MacWeeney, the medical inspector in charge of tuberculosis and of Frank Dowling, a young assistant principal with experience and a wise head on his shoulders, I drew up a plan for TB for the country and presented it to my chiefs in the Department.

Before they had time even to look at it, much less to do anything about it, Professor Theo Dillon, Dan O'Donovan and Dr Harry Counihan, representing the Irish Red Cross, came into the Department and submitted a pilot scheme for the control of tuberculosis to be organised by the Red Cross and carried out on a long-term basis in Dun Laoghaire, a cross-channel port and dormitory town for Dublin. Dun Laoghaire was obviously unsuitable for such a project, being an up-market area with a large population of retired people. Further, we could not wait for a long-term project to show results so I turned it down. In the heated argument with Professor Dillon that followed, I let go and more or less committed the government to ending tuberculosis. This rash promise was leaked to the papers. There was quite a row about it, as being only a civil servant I had no authority to commit the government to a major enterprise like this. However the Department's plan was ready, Mr MacEntee sold it to the Cabinet and I was told to go ahead. Most of the Cabinet were secretly pleased, as I heard afterwards, since in Ireland TB at that time was dreaded. So many families had experience of the disease that they were glad that something was being done about it. In fact some of them had children or relatives of their own suffering from the condition. The programme was published as a White Paper, *Tuberculosis*, in January 1946.

One element of the plan consisted of a short-term programme for the rapid provision of 2,000 additional tuberculosis beds and the longer-term construction of 1,600 beds in
four regional sanatoria. This was based on an overall estimate
of 2.5 beds required per death, including both the existing and
the additional beds. The supply in 1943 amounted to 0.72
beds per death. The bed provision was part of an overall
scheme for prevention and treatment. Actually I did not
regard the details of the plan as being of any great significance,
save as something to sell and to enable us to have an instrument through which we could mobilise people, money and
materials and so get started.

The short-term programme utilised empty fever hospital
beds now no longer required, military hospital beds, beds in
institutions not functioning to full capacity, district hospital
beds and beds in institutions already existing and which
could carry an additional number of patients. We grabbed
beds in places like the new block of ninety beds in Monaghan
Mental Hospital which had been completed as the war began,
but had never been opened.

It became a kind of game to find beds; everybody entered
into the spirit of the thing and Dr Ward gave us tremendous
backing, wielding the big stick to overcome opposition from
people who did not want to part with empty beds or who
were afraid to take on the job of looking after TB patients.
We took over disused military huts and put them in the grounds
of existing institutions. Existing sanatoria were refurbished
as well as possible under war-time conditions and some really
bad accommodation was discontinued.

The long-term programme included three regional sanatoria
and one sub-regional one. Each was to have a central hospital
unit, containing 15/20 per cent of the total beds, while the
remainder of the patients would be housed in forty-bed pavilion blocks.

These blocks were of light construction with a life-expec-
tancy of fifty years and would be available for a variety of
purposes when TB was finally eradicated. Forty beds was
thought to be the optimum number of long-stay patients
which one nursing unit under a Sister could manage. It was
hoped to provide a homely atmosphere in a pleasant situation

with lawns, trees and flowers. Something closer to Irish traditions and psychology than skyscraper tower-blocks. Anyway
we could not get enough steel in the immediate post-war
period to build anything very elaborate. The forty-bed block
was an idea of mine and I did a schedule and a kind of sketch
plan of the thing, but it was Norman White and Mick Jordan
who worked out proper plans and who made them a reality.
We built them for £600 a bed.

The building programme was carried out by a committee
chaired by Ted Courtney, the Chief Engineer of the Department, with Norman White the Chief Architect, Michael Jordan
the Chief Services Engineer, Frank Dowling and myself.

There were all kinds of estimates floating about on the
number of beds needed. These ranged from 4 beds per death
down to 1. I selected a ratio of 2.5 and this was accepted by
the government as a reasonable compromise. I must confess
after all these years that I advanced this figure with tongue in
cheek. The death rates from tuberculosis always rise during a
war. Once the war is over they fall again so current death
rates were misleading. On the other hand we needed enough
if we were to do the job and I felt this was the maximum I
could get away with.

People became obsessed with 'beds', but I believed that they
were only part of an overall public health campaign. Therefore I viewed with a certain amount of dismay the excesses
of enthusiasm for the providing of beds. We had a file called
'Country Mansions', nearly a foot thick, of useless castles and
mansions offered to us as sanatoria with corresponding pressure put on Ministers and other politicians to buy them.

Difficulties in securing the sites were overcome by an Act
pushed quickly through the Dáil by Dr Ward, called the Tuberculosis (Establishment of Sanatoria) Act 1945. This enabled
us to acquire compulsorily any piece of land suitable for a
sanatorium. It remained valid for two years. Looking back on
it, it was probably completely unconstitutional, but such was
the fear of tuberculosis and the relative panic of the times that
we got away with it and no one challenged us.

This business of sites for Regional Sanatoria was interesting.
Sometimes they came easily. For example, one day I was
invited to the Annual Meeting of the Council of the County

Councils. It was followed by a luncheon in the Gresham Hotel and I found myself sitting beside the Mayor of Waterford. Alderman Jones and another Waterford Alderman, whose name I have forgotten, but he was a pig-dealer from Ballybricken, which in my book represents a person with superior intelligence. We were discussing Waterford and I happened to hear them say that Archie de Bromhead was selling his place. I asked them what kind of place it was and they said that it was one of the old Malcomson houses with 60 acres of land and was situated on a bluff above the river and was next to Power's nursery just on the edge of the city. These Malcomson houses had been built in the last century on wonderful sites. The Malcomsons had been great traders and imported cotton from the southern states of America and wove it into quality cloth. During the war between the States, they lent a lot of money to the Confederates which was not repaid and this led to their decline.

The next day I packed the children into my little Ford car and started for Ring, near Waterford, where they were to learn Irish in the famous school run by *An Fear Mor*. Coming back through Waterford I called on Mr de Bromhead. I found that his place was a perfect situation for our new institution and offered to buy it. The next morning I went into Dr Ward, told him what I had done, was scolded a little bit for such an irregularity, but he was quite pleased and the deal was then processed through the proper channels. So that was how we got Ardkeen. You could do things like that in those days.

Galway was a bit more difficult. There was a beautiful 80 acre estate on the edge of the town, called Mervue. It belonged to a Colonel Pierce Joyce, a very interesting person. He was a huge man, a soldier of fortune, having served in many different armies. At one time he had drilled the Arab levies and trained them for the war in the desert when they were led by Lawrence of Arabia. Without Joyce, Lawrence could never have done what he did.

Anyway, with J.D. MacCormack and Theo MacWeeney I went down to Galway to have a look at the place. After a bit, J.D. found himself in the library trying to improve Pierce Joyce's golf swing. Theo was in the drawing room taking tea with Mrs Joyce, a charming old military lady and discussing mutual friends from hill stations in India and elsewhere. Meanwhile I was up on the roof of this great old house, with a sketch pad sketching how we could place or fit in our 40-bed pavilion blocks for the new sanatorium. We concluded by making a tentative offer to buy the place.

Then the fun started. A few days later I had a visit from a Father Kerr, the Provincial of the Redemptorist Order. He was a Belfast man and the son of a very rich and famous solicitor and we knew one another. With his inheritance Father Kerr built a House of Studies to accommodate the young Redemptorist seminarians who were students at Galway University. It was the apple of his eye and here were we coming to build a great sanatorium alongside, since his boundary marched with Mervue. This was intolerable; we would have to move. Firstly, there was the question of infection, though I told him this was nonsense. Then there was the disturbance likely to come from noise, but he was told that as his students were being trained for the missions in the Philippines that it would do them no harm as they would hear a lot of noise when they got to their mission stations. Then there was the question of beautiful young nurses flaunting themselves in the face of the young seminarians steeling themselves to preserve their celibacy and he was told to put opaque glass in the windows facing the sanatorium.

But Father Kerr was not beaten, for who should suddenly turn up in Ireland, all the way from New York, but Father Wainwright, de Valera's half-brother, a member of the Redemptorist Order. Once I heard this I knew that we had had it. So I was sent back to Galway to try again.

I found myself wandering around a place called Merlyn Park, a beautiful estate a couple of miles from Galway on the main Dublin Road. As I wandered through the woods I heard the odd shot and eventually I made my way to the house and, trying to find someone, ended up in the stableyard. A gentleman who had been out shooting was washing his wellingtons at a pump, saw me and asked who I was and what I wanted. When I told him he turned pale and for a moment I thought that he was going to shoot me. He brought me into the house and introduced me to his wife. His name was Wyndham-Waithman and the family had owned the property for many generations. I explained about the establishment of sanatoria Act, but then sat down to present my case and to talk it over with them. I said that we had to have a regional institution in Galway, that I had hunted the area, that we had been displaced from Mervue and that this was the only place left where we could find room for a large institution. As I went on, the enormity of what I was doing, taking their home from these people, became apparent to me. I would like to record the extraordinary christian charity of those two fine people. They agreed that in the face of the terrible problem of tuberculosis in the country, no sacrifice was too much for people to make. They told me to go ahead. It was heart-breaking but there was nowhere else.

Cork was amusing. There it was obviously going to be difficult as the chance of securing a large and suitable area of land near the City was most unlikely. We engaged a local architect, Mr Boyd-Barret, to find us a site and when he had earmarked half-a-dozen places, Ted Courtney, Norman White and I went down to look at them, driven by Dan O'Herlihy, one of Ted's engineers.

We spent three days there wandering around and the sites were all unsuitable and there did not seem anything else in prospect. The next morning we started back for Dublin. As we came around the bend at the end of the river valley at Glanmire I happened to look up and called in a very excited fashion, 'Look fellows, there's our site!' It was Sarsfield Court, one of the most beautiful places in Ireland. It was sitting on a lovely slight slope looking down on the valley and with a background of old trees. We went up and took a look and when Dr Ward heard our description of it the next day he took me down and we bought it from the Hall family, the owners.

From 1945 different parts of the tuberculosis plan were implemented. The plan was constantly improved and fresh things were added. Under Dr Ward and Mr MacEntee we reorganised the x-ray services. Radiologists were appointed, additional equipment purchased as soon as it could be got and free x-ray facilities were made available to all practitioners for the diagnosis and care of tuberculosis. Later chest surgery facilities were provided at six centres which were fully staffed and equipped. Under the Infectious Disease (Maintenance

Regulations) Act of 1947, cash allowances were paid to patients suffering from tuberculosis and to their dependants. Rent allowances, mortgage assistance, clothing, footwear, beds and bedding were provided. Chalets and extra rooms for houses were supplied. Food such as eggs, milk and butter was made available and preferential allocation of local authority housing was given to TB patients and their families.

Rockefeller Fellowship

In the spring of 1946 I was invited to go to London to meet with some of the heads of the Rockefeller Foundation. Since the Lurgan days they had kept in touch with me. They discussed the things we had done in the Custom House and then offered me a Fellowship to America to last two years. When I got back to Dublin and discussed it with Mr MacEntee and Dr Ward it was clear that two years was out of the question in view of our programme, but decent enough they let me go for six months, the Fellowship to commence immediately.

It was a wonderful experience. To be suddenly lifted out of the tension, war-time difficulties and the sometimes non-sensical atmosphere of the Custom House and the Irish health scene was a delight.

In most of the places I visited I was asked to lecture. I would find in a room off the lecture theatre, that they had made available from the library all my published papers, ready so that I could consult them — a pleasant sort of compliment. My travels took me up and down the eastern seaboard of the US and up to Canada. In the University of Toronto I met the people in the Connaught Laboratories and struck up a friendship with them and was so impressed with their work that I arranged that in future they would supply us with 'biologicals' for immunisation and so on. This was of double benefit since materials were hard to come by in those days, particularly supplies which were dependable. On our side we were good customers. So, over the years we had a very successful partnership and a good relationship. J.D. MacCormack visited them later and their people came to see us and studied our needs. On one occasion later when there was a world smallpox scare and certain governments were putting pressure on them for supplies, we found out that they had turned down requests in order to maintain reserve stocks for the Irish government.

Most of my travels were spent in the company of K.A. Jensen, the Director of the State Serum Institute in Copenhagen and a world authority on the manufacture and use of BCG and even more important for the Americans, of penicillin. The Americans were anxious to learn from him and even from me. Everywhere I went I was asked about our programmes, what we were trying to do, what we had managed to achieve, our ideas, about our Infant Mortality Survey in Belfast and about my work in Lurgan and so on. I spent time in the Surgeon-General's office where they were at the beginning of their work in devising a health service for the US, one that met the same kind of fate as ours. They were interested in what we had come up with, how we proposed to finance it and particularly in the preventive approach in general practice and in the development of specialist services.

Wherever I went I asked the question, 'What do you know about enteritis in infants?' Apart from Wayne University in Michigan the answers were the same as we had reached at home. There they had become interested in a virus cause of the condition and agreed to cooperate with us in a study. Park, the great paediatrician in the Johns Hopkins University in Baltimore, had just started the practice of 'cubicalising' infants in Hospital and to use 'barrier' nursing to prevent the spread of infection. Their enteritis was nowhere as widespread or virulent as ours. Park was interested in my *cordon sanitaire*, where we were endeavouring to carry out on a citywide scale more or less what he was doing in his hospital wards.

During this trip I made another kind of advance. So far in my career I had been a general practitioner who ran a practice, did some simple research which in an unusual way had been 'on the ball', was in the Department at the national level, with responsibility but without real authority save for what I could get away with and up till then, the concept of 'high level generalist' had not been thought of. So that when in America people asked me politely, 'What is your field?', they got a different answer every time because I had so many fields that there was no one that I could really claim.

Suddenly I found myself mixing with wonderful people who called themselves 'Public Health' men or women. I found that they had great pride in this designation, that they considered themselves the salt of the earth, they were the people who got things done, the organisers and the people who made things happen. Compared to the clinical people and even the laboratory or the medical teaching folk they were poor, but they had great lives and theirs was an occupation of excitement and happenings. I found that they accepted me as one of themselves and from then on I knew that I too was a 'Public Health' man and nothing else. It was a great feeling to belong and to know that I had finally found my proper 'field'.

6

Irish Hospitals

The hospital situation in Ireland was unique. Outside of Dublin the grand juries, that is to say county committees of ruling Anglo-Irish landlords, had built a series of county infirmaries after 1765. They appointed the surgeons and the accommodation was mainly for themselves, their retainers and people like that. For the vast bulk of the ordinary Irish people there was nothing.

In Dublin there were three medical schools, ten general hospitals classed as teaching hospitals plus others considered as general but not teaching. There were three large lying-in hospitals, three children's hospitals, two specialist hospitals for infectious diseases (fever hospitals), two cancer hospitals and in addition specialist hospitals for eye, ear, nose and throat, dental, orthopaedic and other conditions. This was in addition to large local authority general, geriatric and tuberculosis institutions. In fact tucked away, here and there, were a great variety of ancient or even fairly recent foundations, all doing their own thing. Many were operated by ageing pressure groups or personalities, some of them doing fairly well, some forgotten, but all existing and costing money.

The hospitals were mostly very old; Jervis Street, the Charitable Infirmary, was built in 1719, Dr Steeven's in 1733, Mercer's in 1734 and even the great St Vincent's was housed in an early eighteenth century nobleman's mansion. By today's standards they were tiny little places but they had great traditions and their elaborate boardrooms were lined with the portraits of former staff, some of whom had been world-famous.

In addition there were Houses of Industry for indigent people, which developed, as in the case of the Richmond, Hardwick and Whitworth, into good hospitals. The religious orders founded great hospitals, like the Mater and St Vincent's. It

was in the latter that Florence Nightingale did her training
and from which the nuns went with her to the Crimean War
and did the actual work. As a landmark there was the magnificent Cork Street Fever Hospital founded by the Quakers and
in its day one of the greatest in Europe.

Apart from a few small hospitals in Cork and ancient places
like the County Infirmary in Waterford, where the name
'Leper Asylum' still appears on the facade, there was nothing
else except workhouses which had become hospitals. These
workhouses came about in the following way. Faced with the
appalling circumstances in the country of poverty, disease
and constant epidemics of cholera, typhus and typhoid, the
Anglo-Irish government decided to apply to Ireland the English
Poor Law System. George Nicholls, an English Poor Law
Commissioner, was sent over to examine the problem and to
report. He was a remarkable man, a workhouse master's son
who knew what he was doing. He rode right around Ireland
in six weeks, talking to everybody including the viceroy, the
tramps, the priests, the landlords and the doctors and quickly
drew up a plan to apply the Poor Law here. This was based
on unions of parishes, to be supervised by Boards of Guardians
and with a Workhouse in each union. The plan was accepted
by Whitehall and the word was given to go ahead. The Ulster
landlords tried to opt out of any such social commitment so
Nicholls came back the following year and said 'No' to them,
they were in it too. Today is not the first time that the leaders
in the north gave meaning to the expression 'Ulster says No'.

The work of building the workhouses began in the early
1840s and the sites were selected by military engineers. They
were built of cut-stone to a common pattern. The buildings
included day rooms, dining halls, a chapel, kitchens, laundries,
schools for children, sick quarters, fever blocks, and in some
cases, separate cholera blocks. Sleeping accommodation was
in long wards with central passages and raised side platforms
on which people lay on straw. The sexes were to be separated
and families broken up.

Work began quickly and a hundred such buildings were
completed by 1845, just before the great Famine broke in
1847. The work was pushed on and by 1850 a further eighty
had been built. They were just in time to save the lives of vast

numbers of the Irish who would otherwise have died of starvation. Considering the times and the circumstances this was
probably the greatest and most effective social institutional
building programme ever completed anywhere.

On the night of the Census of March 1851 the number of
people behind workhouse walls for food and shelter was
249,000. In two years more than one million people were
admitted and received food, shelter and clothing from these
institutions. On one day in July 1847 from a total population
of about eight millions, three millions received free food. In
the fever hospitals in 1847 and 1848 more than 275,000 were
admitted each year. In six years more than a million people
emigrated. The Deenys have an interest in these workhouses
because my great-grandfather, Michael Deeny, a gaelic scholar
and a master-mason from the Sperrin Mountains, worked on
the building of Carndonagh workhouse in Donegal. The money
earned there probably saved his family from starvation.

These places eventually became a hospital system for the
country. Not a hospital system as we know it but a place where
sick people could go when they had nowhere else. Here and
there, when Boards of Guardians had money, they were
improved. The credit for this was more often than not due to
the local medical officers of the workhouses. They demanded
better conditions for the people and nearly everywhere there
was a constant battle between the Boards of Guardians who
were concerned with the cost and the medical officers whose
anxiety was human welfare.

I knew about workhouses since during my summer holidays
in Lurgan, in one of these 'improved' hospitals, Dr Darling
the surgeon allowed me to assist him as a medical student with
his enormous operation lists. Later when I came to Dublin I
found here and there in the country some workhouse hospitals
which had changed very little. In Longford there were still
'twelve-holer' earth closets.

Sometime in 1922-23, shortly after the establishment of
the Department of Local Government and Public Health, an
official instruction was issued to the local IRA leaders (before
the new Free State services were properly functioning) to
remove the old people from all the workhouses and bring them
to one centre in each county which from then on was desig-

nated as the County Home.

The empty workhouses soon became derelict or were turned into district hospitals. The transfer could only have been done in this way, practically at the point of the gun. Otherwise, local influences and interests would never have allowed the closure of local institutions, no matter how inadequate. The Government, up to the outbreak of war, had constructed more than 40 hospitals. However, they needed a planned modern health service in which the hospitals would act as units and centres for specialist services which up to this time did not exist. My job was to plan this.

With the coming of the Sweepstakes, the Hospitals Commission was established to advise on the construction and reconstruction of the hospital system. The Department gradually took over the planning and the building of the hospitals. In the building of a hospital we followed a fixed procedure. We had a list of priorities which we had drawn up and which depended on the needs of areas, the state of existing institutions in the hierarchal hospital structure. We might put up a proposal for consideration that such and such a place should have a new hospital and this would be examined by the administrators and then would go to the Minister for approval.

More often than not the Minister would also have his priorities. He would be under pressure from party members to build a hospital here or there for this or that reason or to satisfy a demand from a local pressure group or interest. He had to keep one eye on the spokesperson on health of the Opposition who was usually very well-informed from his local supporters, either political or in various strata of the health professions. Then in his own party there might be amateur or professional 'authorities' who had to be treated carefully.

Most Ministers of Health are fully conscious of the 'pork-barrel' effect of a new hospital in the community on jobs, contracts and prestige. On the other hand there is the question, 'Do you really need a hospital?' 'Will it become a heavy burden on the tax-payers of the future?' 'Can you down-face the technical advice of your staff?'

If the Minister gave approval we went ahead. If he did not then the proposal might travel around the Department being 'examined' or repose on someone's desk while we got on with something else or the Government changed or whatever. If the proposal was to go ahead the matter was conveyed to the local authority, usually the County Council, or possibly a religious order. They then appointed an architect.

During my time as CMA in the Department I would then do the Outline Schedule. This laid out what the hospital would do, the various units it would need to do it, the size of the place in terms of beds, an idea of the staffing and the equipment needed, usually in broad terms. I would attempt to place it in the hospital hierarchy and its relationship with other institutions. This would then have to be accepted by the Minister and all around the Department.

Then it would go to Charlie Lysaght, who later succeeded me, and who became one of the greatest hospital building experts in Europe, because he had built more hospitals than anyone else. Charlie would meet with the locally appointed architects and with our own equally experienced architectural staff, who were highly skilled and expert. They would plan the Detailed Schedule and would work on it. The local authority architect would study this further and consult the local doctors and would then come up with a sketch plan. This would be shown around, possibly a model would be made, and the local authority people would all have their say. For example someone would want a 'cut-stone' job from a certain quarry, very reasonably because it would mean local employment. All kinds of other local interests might emerge. Then it would go a stage further with the Lay-Out Plan, the circulation of people in the hospital, the services necessary such as electricity, piped oxygen, the relationship of one unit to another, things like kitchens to wards and dining rooms, the fuel to be used, heating, sanitation and a hundred other different factors were considered. All this meant continual discussion, considerations of plans, the introduction of new technology and hundreds of different features, all needing to be studied. Finally there were the Working Drawings and then the quantity surveyors came in and 'took-out' the material requirements needed to build the hospital, down to the last nail and the last can of paint.

Our colleagues on the administrative side were concerned with such matters as the purchase of sites, tenders and contracts, finance, purchasing of equipment, the personnel side of staffing and a very large segment of the task which could be regarded as administrative as opposed to technical. It is important to emphasise the administrative aspect since it is easy to become very extravagant in the building of a hospital. Equally the administrative people had to have a certain responsibility in that cheese-paring could ruin a hospital. To cut a foot off the width of all corridors might save a great deal of money but it might mean darkness, cramped conditions, difficulty in handling trolleys and misery in the running of the hospital. Equally 'waste space' is waste in terms of heating, lighting, cleansing, noise and dozens of foolish nonsenses, often tributes to someone's vanity.

In our 1945 plan we had envisaged five hospital groupings for Dublin. An enlarged Mater and a new hospital on the north-side, the present Beaumont. We wanted a new St Vincent's at Elm Park and the site had already been purchased by the Irish Sisters of Charity. We intended to use the vast complex of St James' hospital, then called St Kevin's, as another centre and then for the large population on the southern coastal strip, there would be St Michael's in Dun Laoghaire and a recon-structed Loughlinstown. We had not foreseen, in 1945, the tremendous extension of the city to the west. Due to a variety of circumstances our progress in Dublin was much slower than in the rest of the country.

One could say that we equalled the people who built the workhouses a hundred years before. Starting with forty county and other new hospitals in place just before the Second World War, as soon as the situation returned to normal and supplies of building materials and hospital equipment became available again, we carried out a formidable programme. We built regional and teaching hospitals, regional sanatoria, mental hospitals, county hospitals, specialist hospitals, clinics, dis-pensaries and other health institutions. In addition we rebuilt, renovated or refurbished many institutions such as county homes and other geriatric accommodation. All-in-all in the years 1940-65, (ten of these being largely inoperative due to the war) more than two hundred hospitals were built and another large number reconstructed, ranging from multi-million pound vast edifices down to small humble county accommodation.

I claim, on behalf of all the people who took part in it, that one of the great achievements of this state since its foundation was the building of the hospitals. They were the first large buildings constructed in Ireland for generations. Few realise what an interesting team job it was. We could commence with the families who founded the Irish Hospital Sweepstakes, the MacGraths, the Duggans and the Freemans, who by their brains and hard work produced the vast bulk of the money to pay for the programme. By selling pieces of paper all over the world, entitling people to become rich overnight, if they were lucky, huge sums became available to pay for the construction of hospitals in Ireland. Then we had a succession of highly intelligent Ministers who laid the foundation of the political side of the business and kept matters under control through bodies like the Hospitals Commission. Nevertheless, to my mind the building of the hospitals was mainly a technical feat. It is to the 'backroom boys', the doctors, architects, contractors, engineers and Irish craftsmen that most of the credit is due. The others played their parts well, participated fully, and performed the official openings nicely, but it was the technical people who counted.

The Westmoreland Lock Hospital

One of the great things about the Custom House was that something interesting turned up almost every day. For instance, sometime early in 1947 I had a visit from a Mr Ross. He said that he was the Secretary of the Lock Hospital and that they were in difficulties. I had never heard of the Lock Hospital and said so. He brought me to a window of my office and pointed to it, just across the river in Townsend Street, a few hundred yards away.

Near the end of the eighteenth century the Anglo-Irish government set up several Houses of Industry. They were places where beggars, indigent sick and other waifs of society could be sent to get them out of sight. They included the present Richmond, Hardwick and Whitworth Hospitals, St James' Hospital and the Westmoreland Lock Hospital, called after the Earl of Westmoreland, the Viceroy of the day. These hospitals were run by Boards of Governors appointed directly by the Viceroy. When the Free State was established an Act was

passed transferring the right of nomination of Governors to
the Minister of Local Government and Public Health. Unfortunately those framing the Act knew nothing about the Lock
and so failed to include it and to give it a legal basis for existing. Mr Ross had been carrying on ever since as best he could,
charging local authorities for the services of the hospital to
patients for whom they were responsible.

Unfortunately for him, his hospital and his patients, the
local authorities had found out that there was no legal compulsion on them to pay and so were refusing to meet his bills.
Also the Board of Governors, last appointed in the British
times, had dwindled down to two survivors, both of whom
were over eighty; one had become paralysed and was bed-ridden
so there was no one available to sign the cheques. Even if there
had been, the bank would not give them any more credit and
they were broke. Faced with this sad situation Mr Ross took
it into his head to come to see me. I took time off and went
with him to have a look at the place.

The Westmoreland Lock Hospital had been founded more
than 200 years before for the treatment of venereal diseases. It
provided 200 beds and an outpatient's department. There
were similar foundations in London and Edinburgh. The hospital was a long, low, quite elegant Georgian building. The
outpatient department had a discreet entrance down a little
side-street. It was the kind of place which the ordinary citizen
might pass daily without ever wondering what went on inside.
However, once inside, it was a revelation.

Although it had beds for 200, only thirty or so were occupied, all by females. These were mainly elderly prostitutes,
although some younger women were there and a few babies
were to be seen. The atmosphere was, to say the least, relaxed
and informal. The ladies were 'taking their ease', having the
odd game of cards, smoking, singing the odd song and con-
suming the odd bottle of Guinness. Mr Ross and the Matron
took me on a tour and showed me the great empty wards. I
saw the dining room where the ladies sat at little marble-
topped tables under a huge portrait of the Earl of Westmoreland, dressed up in his robes as a Knight of the Garter and
looking down on them with an eighteenth century leer. There
had been formerly a strict segregation of the patients by

religion. There was a Catholic chapel and a Protestant church. To reach the church one traversed a long dark corridor, illuminated only by a door with stained glass at the far end. This had a text in ruby glass which read, 'Even though my sins are scarlet, they shall be washed white as snow'. The basement had a long beautifully vaulted corridor with rooms off and the kitchen was feudal.

I was shown the house rules which had been drawn up about 200 years ago. They were quaint but of an undreamt-of harshness. Possibly the most lenient was the punishment to be exacted on women who exposed themselves from the windows. There were severe penalties for patients who had a pin in their clothes lest they infect the doctors from a scratch when they were being examined. Nurses also got into trouble for this. Up on the roof, in a kind of wooden tower, there was a special chamber where syphilitics inhaled mercury fumes. I think the old time doctors felt that the patients had had enough when their teeth fell out. In the basement I saw rooms like dungeons where they kept people suffering from general paralysis of the insane, a sequela of syphilis, in which people became megalomaniac and often violent. There was a story that at one time they maintained a military guard over such patients as there were so many of them and they were so dangerous.

Clearly we had to do something about this, so Dr Ward introduced a Bill to regularise things and at the same time we looked for additional powers to enable us to do more for venereal disease. We appointed a specialist VD officer for the city and got a good one in Dr Lanigan-O'Keefe. We started other clinics and I remember the Archbishop being very helpful when we proposed one for the Mater Hospital. Anyway, we got an organised service going.

Mr Ross, having done his duty by the place, retired shortly after and, as Dr Stirling Berry from the Department was about to retire and was anxious for something to do, he was appointed to take the place over. With Berry in charge, a new Board, some money to spend, this terrible old place was transformed.

As part of the improvements the Governors thought that if the ladies learnt cooking and housekeeping they might be rehabilitated and find jobs. After a lot of difficulty finding someone willing to take them on we dug up a retired home economics teacher, an old saint. On the occasion of the first lesson, the Matron, who was quite excited about this new venture, invited the Board to visit the classroom. The Board descended in processional order to the basement and proceeded along the corridor to where a room had been fixed up as a classroom. When we entered we found our ladies all sitting primly at desks in nice new pinafore aprons and on a large blackboard was the first lesson. It was 'Bachelor Pudding'. The Board dissolved in a *fou-de-rire* and ran for their lives, but actually this effort worked. In spite of all, human goodness was still there in this dreadful place. The Matron was a remarkable person. She mothered and cared for these poor women and her goodness had a wonderful effect on them. On one occasion when she became very ill the inmates would not let her go to hospital and two former patients who had reformed and had become nurses gave up good jobs in London, came back, nursed her and never left her bedside till she recovered.

Baggot Street Hospital
One of the problems on my mind was the provision of decent health services for the great new housing estates which Dublin Corporation and private builders had created all around the old city.

We had the usual poor law dispensaries and in one way they gave a good service to the limited areas in their immediate surroundings. They were only open for a few hours a day and not every day and there were few if any practitioners living on these estates. A few doctors lived on the outskirts of the areas. Many families had as a tradition always attended the outpatients clinic of some hospital or other but now that they had been rehoused it was a long and inconvenient trek for them to go to receive medical care. Even to this day it seems that the problem has not been solved.

I tried in 1947 to do something about this problem but met with little success. It happened this way. Baggot Street Hospital, otherwise known as The Royal City of Dublin Hospital, wanted to build a new outpatient's clinic and applied to the Minister for the money. This was an interesting little hospital which had been founded by a group of doctors about a hundred years before and was still owned by their successors.

I found that the prime space of the hospital on the mezzanine was taken up by students' quarters (including a large billiard room), the Matron's parlour, where she dispensed coffee to the senior staff each morning, and an elaborate Board room. The really essential area of the hospital was taken up with these pleasant amenities. The site where they proposed to put the new outpatients was really the backyard of the hospital and was anyway too cramped. They wanted £50,000, which at that time was a lot of money.

I came back with a counter-proposal which was that we would build them a clinic at Crumlin, a housing estate with a population of more than 40,000 people at that time. We planned to link it with the existing Poor Law dispensary. This would mean that in addition to the existing general practitioner service we would have specialist services provided by the hospital in sessions staffed by the senior registrars. The idea was experimental and if it worked well we could extend it to other hospitals and so could cover all the conurbations. As a carrot I said that we would pay the registrars, who at that time and in those hospitals had only a very thin living.

I never realised what a hornet's nest I had stirred up and to this day do not know why the senior hospital staff would not have it. Decent old men, senior physicians, cut me dead. They came on deputations to the Minister, they lobbied all over the place and because they had a lot of 'clout' and fought every inch of the way, the word got around to other hospitals and opposition grew. So I threw my hat at it and they won. It was not worth all the trouble and Dublin would have to wait. In the end they got their way and spent the £50,000 in their backyard.

County Homes

The Congregation of the Sisters of Mercy was founded in 1827 by Mother Catherine MacAuley. Later she had the idea that the sisters would go into the workhouses and try to improve the lot of people condemned to these places. At the time it was a most enlightened idea. The Catherine MacAuleys, the Nano Nagles, Aikenheads and the founders of such orders were the Mother Theresas of their day.

When I started to visit the County Homes shortly after I

was appointed I found women, some of them old, who thirty
or forty years before had been unmarried mothers, were disowned by their families and had fetched up for shelter in the
workhouse. They had been assigned to work in the kitchen or
laundry as being 'able-bodied female paupers'. They had spent
years or even a lifetime working without pay, dressed up in
the workhouse garb, literally slaves. In the kitchens, unchanged
for a hundred years, one could see great cauldrons into which
metal baskets containing hundred-weights of potatoes were
lowered by small cranes to boil for the inmates' dinners. These
were quite unprotected and the odd old woman might fall in
and be roasted.

During the war maintenance had fallen off, spouts were
broken, windows not repaired or any painting carried out,
not even white-washing. To visit some of these places on a
damp day and feel the humidity, see the water streaming down
the walls and sense the cold, the musty workhouse smell and
the depression, misery and hopelessness there, was grim.

These things were all part of an era which, thank God, was
nearing its end and I was just in time to say goodbye to it. But
I saw what it was like. The paupers were the forgotten people
of the old Ireland. They included elderly farm-labourers who,
as was customary in parts of the country, had spent a lifetime
sleeping in byres. Wizened little men, such as I had seen as a
boy riding strings of horses from one horse fair to another.
Old women farm servants, thrown out when they were past
work, and other categories of poor 'done' people. In Dublin
there were prim elderly maids from Ballsbridge and Donny-
brook who had served for a lifetime but were now forgotten
and homeless with the protestant wards in St Kevin's as their
only refuge. There were old unmarried uncles who had become
a nuisance, grocer's 'curates' who had become alcoholics,
unmarried old women without support, a vast horde of old
people, many crippled with arthritis, often demented through
malnutrition and hardship, lonely, miserable and hungry. The
workhouse was the only place which would take them.

To see a poor old man just admitted and given a bowl of
milk and rice and to see him lift it to his face and devour it
like a dog, shook you, because you suddenly realised that he
was starving. In the new Ireland, no matter how much we

complain, no matter how badly we feel that things are not good enough, we have created a better world for the old people certainly compared with what existed a generation or so ago.

But in Ireland things are never all bad. You might walk into such a ward and find an old man dying and all the other old men, his mates, praying out aloud, praying him into Heaven. Meanwhile a nun held his hand, talking to him and helping him on his way with love and kindness.

Amongst the matrons there was one in Mountmellick whom I remember with admiration. On my way to Dublin one night I dropped in to have a look at the place and found her doing her night round. She tucked all the old men in and said good-night to them, just as if they were babies. One old chap had the bedclothes over his head but held one arm out rigidly above his bed. When she came to him she squeezed his hand and put it under the clothes and only then would he go to sleep. This was a nightly ritual.

This matron got fed up with her old men spending their pensions on the town, for if they had too much to drink and tried to make their way back to the home they could fall into a puddle of rain and if the search party did not locate them in time they might die there or at least get pneumonia by morning. So she started a bar. She took a half-penny profit from each bottle of stout she sold and re-invested her profits in things like electric razors or anything the old fellows wanted. This was really an illegal shebeen and she was scared lest I should find it. I saw the electric razors hanging up and asked where did she get them, as forty years ago they were unusual in workhouses for paupers. So she confessed and I must admit I encouraged her in her criminal ways.

7

The New Department of Health and its Ministers

In 1947 a separate Department of Health was established. It was badly needed and without it we could never have achieved what we did. From the medical side's point of view one of the most important things to happen was that we received an influx of new staff such as Harry O'Flanagan, Tom Murphy, Michael Daly, Gus Jennings, Malachy Powell, Tim Murphy and Jerry O'Sullivan. They had varied experience, a multitude of talents, had a common dedication to the work and enormous energy.

We began a slow improvement in our relations with the medical profession all over the country. As the medical inspections resumed after the war we also developed satisfactory working arrangements with the great numbers of local authority staffs of the county and city councils. So great was our programme that the existing medical team was very hard pressed and the addition of a new young active group was a blessing.

At the same time the establishment of the new Department brought into the health field new young administrators. This lot included some of the ablest young men in the civil service, who were attracted to the new Department by the promise of action, by a sense of compassion and by the interesting things going on. They included some seniors like Padraic O'Cinneide, who had been assistant secretary in the Department of the Taoiseach and who became the first Secretary of the Department, in addition to a string of youngsters who are today's heads of the Department. Most of the nice old men, whom we liked and respected so much, stayed within the relatively safe confines of the Department of Local Government.

It was a highly successful foundation. In a sense it contrasted well with the Department of Social Welfare, set up at

about the same time. John Garvin and I, representing the
Department of Local Government and Public Health, were
members of the Inter-Departmental Committee set up to consider the establishment of a Department of Social Welfare.
Louis Fitzgerald of the Department of Finance was chairman.
Up to that time social welfare in Ireland consisted of a number
of schemes administered by different Departments and this
did not make sense. For instance, the children's allowance
scheme was for some reason in the hands of the Department
of Industry and Commerce with a staff of over one hundred
people under an Assistant Secretary to run it.

Each member of the committee had come to dump a part
of the social services which he administered and which he
wished to be rid of on to the new Department. A package of
these services was put together, neatly parcelled up into a new
Department of State and that was that, a neat administrative
job. John Garvin and I did not like this and so we wrote a
Minority Report. So far as I can remember we pointed out
that without legs and arms to do things, economically and
socially, and without a research and development brain, it
would never be anything other than a 'dole-paying' agency,
which in fact it became. Our Minority Report fell flat on its
face and nothing happened. I heard on the grape-vine that
from time to time Lemass and other ministers would take it
down from its pigeon-hole, dust it off and read it, but nothing
happened and it was always consigned again to its forty-year
slumber.

In May 1948 the first assembly of the World Health Organisation took place in Geneva and with J.D. MacCormack and Tom
Brady I attended. Because of our neutrality it was the only
new UN Agency to which Ireland was invited. It was one of
the proudest moments of my life when I marched up to the
rostrum as the Chief of the Irish Delegation to enter our
appearance. On the way up, ringing in my ears was Robert
Emmet's speech from the dock, in Green Street Courthouse
in Dublin, when he was condemned to death and when he
said: 'Not till my country takes its place amongst the nations
of the Earth, is my epitaph to be written'. Here was Ireland
taking its place and I had the honour of representing it, truly
an emotional and moving experience. This had probably an

influence on the next episode.

While the three of us were sitting in our places waiting for the game to begin, Sir Wilson Jameson, the Chief Medical Officer of the Ministry of Health of England came by and he said, 'James, let me present the UK Delegation'. There were present Melville MacKenzie, Buchanan, Sandy Rae, and Hector Lindsay. Jameson was a very good friend of mine, whom I admired and respected, but I could not contain myself and asked, 'Where's Davidson? (CMO Scotland).' Jameson said, 'James, aren't five Scotsmen enough to represent the United Kingdom?' and I replied, 'No! Scotland is a nation as old as the earth and her Chief should be here.' He gave a snort and marched on at the head of his men. But the following year Davidson came and he, and in after years his successors, thanked me for that remark. Neither Wales or the North of Ireland ever made it to the assembly, at least not in my time.

One of the conclusions from the first assembly was that I had a lot of things to attend to at home. Another was that J.D. was so popular, and so good at the job, that he would represent Ireland very much better than I would and that it was better that he should carry on. So for years I attended the assembly on very few occasions and stayed at home to mind the shop.

When the county inspections were resumed we altered the nature of the task. For nearly a century the job of the inspectors was, say in a dispensary, to check the records kept by the doctor of his attendances and visits against the number of 'tickets' which the patients were supposed to present before the doctor rendered a service. The stock of drugs was inspected and the equipment of the dispensary examined. Finally the state of the dispensary and the midwife services and other things were all dealt with and the whole made into a report which came up to the CMA in the Department for examination. If any action was required he sent it along to the administrative side for attention.

I was anxious to change the approach of the inspectors. In future their role should be to try to improve the service any way they could. They should try to work with the doctor whom they were inspecting. They should help to solve problems, to provide a 'pipe-line' for the doctor to the Department, to discuss policy and to try to do a constructive job. They were expected to establish good relations with the medical profession in the counties for which they were responsible.

In the past medical inspectors remained in their districts for weeks on end. Files and instructions for the attention of the inspectors were sent to them in locked dispatch cases which were carried by the hotel porters to and from the railway stations. There was a collection system from the Custom House at the other end when all mail trains were met and the dispatch bags taken in a van to headquarters. For years I wondered at the item of two shillings under the heading of 'porterage' which appeared always and invariably on the expense sheets of the inspectors until I found out that this was the tip given to the hotel porters for their trouble in handling the dispatch cases.

The inspectors were judged by the amount of work they turned in and in one sense this was a good system and of value in that they spent a lot of their time in their districts and came to know everybody and everything that was going on. On the other hand their family lives suffered as they wandered around from hotel to hotel, often lonely and miserable.

I changed the protocol and brought them back to Dublin each week-end. Of course their work did not suffer and they were happier people. We also had a staff meeting every Saturday morning. This was before the introduction of a five-day working week. One of the group would make a presentation at the meeting. This would be on some topical subject or problem and then we would have a discussion. When we had finished this we would have a free-for-all discussion. These talks were hilarious. Sometimes the group told me what they thought of me, very bluntly and not always very politely. Equally I would get mad at them and tell them what I thought of their shortcomings. What is described in today's diplomatic language as a 'useful exchange of views'. But the real pleasure was that every eccentricity, every funny story, every joke and hoax in the country found its way back to my room in the Custom House. The roars of laughter on a Saturday morning used to shake the dome of the Custom House because, after all, Ireland is a very funny country and Irish people have not only a great enjoyment of folly but a constant healthy need to laugh at themselves and everybody else. The noise was so great that on one occasion Mr MacEntee, who was receiving a delegation from the Workers' Union of Ireland, sent his private secretary around to tell us 'for God's sake to keep quiet', that we could be heard all over the building and that we were embarrassing him in the matter of the delicate negotiations he was conducting. The secretary ran for his life when the group collectively gave him a rude message to carry back to the Minister and to the Union.

This weekly return to base enabled the field men to consult with and receive advice from their older colleagues, to meet one another and exchange views and to secure backing for a particular line of action or whatever. It also became important to us that we should have a professional forum and this we achieved. The state medicine section of the Royal Academy of Medicine was pretty well moribund and had few meetings of any interest and a very small attendance. We moved in on this, organised good meetings with papers of topical interest, brought our interesting visitors along to speak and soon it was the second-best attended of all the many sections of the Academy. For a public health forum, which the clinicians usually regarded as dull, it was quite an achievement. This was of great value because we needed a place where we could meet on a professional basis with our peers, present our ideas, have them criticised by people who knew what they were talking about and have decent honest arguments about things. There was an additional satisfaction in that we had visits from people all over the world. They came to see what we were doing since the word had got about that things were happening here.

For the first few years of my service in the Department, life was fine. It was exceedingly hard work and required constant attention to keep all the irons I had in the fire nice and hot. On the other hand, once a thing was moving my colleagues really did the work. What was often an idea in my mind and a half-baked scheme sold to a Minister became in their hands a fully effective project and more importantly, was punched through to a successful completion.

As they pass into history it is worth writing something about the Ministers as I remember them. One should appreciate that the first few people I worked for were men who in their time had been revolutionaries, had faced death or been imprisoned. Whatever they got up to in the Dáil, in the Department they were very much in earnest.

My first chiefs were Dr Con Ward and Mr Sean MacEntee, with Con Ward as Parliamentary Secretary in charge of Health and MacEntee as the Minister of Local Government and Public Health.

Con Ward had been a very successful practitioner and dispensary doctor in the town of Monaghan. Although he had lived and practised only forty miles or so from me in Lurgan, I had never met him. Because of the border Monaghan was on the other side of the moon but I was aware of his reputation as a first-class doctor. He had a strong background in the old IRA and formerly had raided for arms all over the counties of Monaghan, Cavan and Tyrone, with occasional forays into the county Armagh. He had a traditional Irish background. One of his brothers was the Prior of Lough Derg, the age-old island pilgrimage in Donegal, the other a senior Christian Brother. He was a formidable, almost hypnotic man and it took courage to stand up to him. He had a remarkable memory and did not suffer fools to indulge in their foolishness. If a delegation came in and some unfortunate made a statement with which Dr Ward did not agree he would call a halt to the proceedings and everyone would sit in embarrassed silence until the file was produced and then Ward with deliberation would read out what was on the file, usually proving the poor character to be in the wrong, rubbing his nose in the dirt and cutting him down to size. This did not endear him to the population at large but that did not worry Ward. Looking back on it I do not altogether blame him. There was so much opposition to everything Fianna Fáil did and so much of it, judged on purely technical grounds, was so unfair that one could forgive him for being tough. On the other hand Fianna Fáil, having tasted power, used it. If you belonged to any other party you could reasonably feel that they were hard to stand. I had a very uneasy relationship with him at first and actually did not properly understand him. Then eventually I blew up, had my strike and made my point. After that I got to know him better, came to respect him, laughed at him first, then with him and finally came to like him very much. He had a delightful family who adored him, and a wonderful wife.

In everything we tried to do once you convinced this hard-headed Monaghan man, who was also a first-class experienced doctor, that the idea was sound you could be assured of his whole-hearted support and backing.

Unfortunately he made enemies in the party. When things started to move and he got credit for them in the newspapers there was jealousy. He had not a lot of personal support as he was too much of a 'loner'. He had also antagonised the medical profession. A former close friend of his, and a former president of the Irish Medical Association, wrote to de Valera, accusing Ward of corruption on fourteen counts, most of them trivial and in connection with a bacon business he had in Monaghan. De Valera promptly proposed a judicial tribunal to examine the affair.

Dr. Ward sent for me and told me the story. After all the fights we had had it was extraordinary that I was the one he turned to. I advised him to resign and to go to the courts with an action for slander. He had a constitutional right to do this. I felt that he would win as the defendant would have to prove his case in open court. With a tribunal he would have to prove his innocence and with fourteen counts, no matter how trivial, it would be next to impossible to do this.

But he was so sure of the outcome and of his ability to clear himself that he accepted the tribunal. For days on end he defended himself in what was an extraordinary legal process, watched by a multitude of enemies who came to gloat. It was the nearest thing to a Stalin trial ever seen in modern Ireland, at least so I thought at the time. The judges cleared him on all counts save one, an income tax irregularity; on this they said that they were not prepared to believe him. So he resigned and went back to his practice in Monaghan. Later if I was in or near there I went to see him. I found him reconciled, serene and extraordinarily happy. In fact I drew strength from seeing someone with such courage in adversity. It was a tragedy that we lost him from the Custom House.

Sean MacEntee, the Minister for Local Government and Health from 1942, was an elegant little man, always beautifully turned out, with most courteous manners, a bon viveur, a cultured intellectual and charming. He was a completely different sort to most of the other Ministers, who were stern, solid types.

MacEntee had a most wicked tongue. During elections he would say the most outrageous things about his political opponents and then would go through agonies of remorse for his cruel taunts. He was completely political; while Con Ward would see a thing from the medical point of view MacEntee only saw the political aspects. He had a first-class brain and was as quick as lightning. The trouble was to prevent him going off half-cock on some idea that he would pick up somewhere and which he would pursue with breathless enthusiasm. However this could be refreshing if it did not get out of hand.

Sean MacEntee more than anyone else put his mark on local government. At one time in Ireland there were more than two hundred and fifty large and small local administrations. Each was a little political battle-ground with every local interest represented, each one blocking the other so that progress was impossible. The system was beautifully independent of control and this was an irritation to central government. MacEntee continued a process begun by some of his predecessors and slimmed the lot down to twenty-six county councils and four county boroughs and developed the managerial system. The local appointments selection system produced efficient managers who soon saw action at the local level.

MacEntee was a perfectionist, something of a poet and was particular about good civil service writing and presentation. He tolerated the famous writer Flann O'Brien (Myles na gCopaleen) for years. He liked to move in elegant circles. His wife was a lecturer in UCD. He was a peppery little man and a bit vain. In an expansive mood I once referred to the Department of Health as 'my Department', as I would refer to Lurgan as 'my town' or to Armagh as 'my county'. He heard of it and I received a little note from him pointing out that the Minister was the only one who could refer to the Department as 'my Department'. However despite such little exhibitions of vanity, I respected him very much and admired his qualities. He had really a lot going for him. When Dr Ward left and the new Department of Health was established in 1947, he was the first Minister. He showed very great compassion and courage in the fight we made to clear up Dublin's child health problem and he supported our efforts to get the TB campaign going. In 1946 he began, almost single-handed, except for the wise advice of Seamas MacNeill the Dental Adviser in the Department, and pushed through a nation-wide fluoridation scheme, which has been of inestimable benefit to the children of this country.

Dr James Ryan, the second Minister of Health, I admired. It was a pleasure to work for him. He was a gentle soul and kind and he too had a first-class brain. The first thing he found on his plate as Minister for Health was a difficult little problem. We had acquired Santry Court, an estate on the main North Road, just outside Dublin, as a site for our new regional sanatorium. It was an 'instant' site as it was owned by the Dublin Corporation and we, the sanatorium committee, just took it. It became famous afterwards as the sports track of the Clonliffe Harriers and the place where for the first time in history, three people cracked the four minute mile, a race I had the good luck to see. Once we had our hands on it, we went ahead very quickly and installed sewers, ducts, water-mains and all kinds of site development work. The work was going along well, when one day a friend of mine in the Department of Finance rang me and asked whether I was aware that a new runway was about to be built at Dublin Airport and that it would end about fifty yards from the boundary of our sanatorium where, of course, peace and quiet would be essential.

The gentlemen sitting around the Cabinet table had taken two decisions. One was to build the runway, the other to build the sanatorium. Both had been communicated to the Secretaries of the Departments concerned, but no one had troubled to connect the two ideas, and tell us, the people who were busily engaged in building this huge sanatorium. Ted Courtney, Norman White and I promptly went in to see MacEntee and I told him the news. He asked us what he should do, saying that de Valera would be within his rights to ask for the resignation of any Minister who had presided over such a gaffe. I said that this was a matter for ministerial decision and would he kindly give us a direction. The next thing was that Ted, Norman and I found ourselves, for most of a freezing night, at the end of the main runway at Shannon airport, taking decibel readings of the noise made by planes taking off for the US and Canada and estimating what it would be like to have to lie in bed and have this going on while you lay sick in our new sanatorium.

We came back and said that it was not on, and that Lemass should go and build his runway somewhere else. Lemass, being Lemass, would not buy this idea, so again we asked for a direction from the Minister. It became a battle of wits, because MacEntee asked constantly for our advice and we came back and said that we could not advise him on the problem and that he should tell us what his decision was. We did not say that it was his mistake and that if it came to a show-down we were not going to carry the can and allow him to say that he had been advised to do so and so. After a couple of weeks of good civil service amusement, he kicked for touch and said that the matter might await the arrival of a new Minister of Health.

The new Minister of Health was Dr Ryan. We put the matter to him immediately. Now if I had been faced with such a problem, particularly as there was a tremendous political heat on about tuberculosis and sanatoria all over the place, it might have upset me, but James Ryan went home, slept the sleep of the just and came in the next morning and told us to get a new site, quietly to stop work on the old one and to say nothing. This was of course just what we had been waiting to hear.

We promptly went out and selected Lord Holmpatrick's place at Abbotstown, bought it, and moved in. I had had my eye on it for some time and the bit of research I had done on it came in handy. Dr Ryan then announced the change in his own quiet way, without any fuss, no one said anything and that was that. They got away with six months delay and £60,000 worth of work underground (a large sum in those days). Doctors are not the only people to bury their mistakes.

One day, I was going to Galway with James Ryan to some official opening of something or other and after passing Athlone, I said that there was someone I wanted him to meet. This was a little man, almost a dwarf, who had a TB spine. The vertebrae had collapsed and he was a hunch-back. His spinal cord had been damaged so that he was paralysed from the waist down. He lived a bit off the main road, but on a good day his family would bring him from his home and set him down on a bank on the side of the road so that he could see what was going on. If I saw him when passing, I used to stop and chat with him, and found that in spite of his handicap, he was a delightful cheery soul. He dearly loved the old chat. This day he was in position and we stopped and I introduced the Minister and stood back and let Dr Ryan and himself at it. He was a witty little man and charmed Dr Ryan. He too was delighted to meet the Minister. Later, when we got into the car and moved off, Dr Ryan said, 'I've always wanted to do something for people like that. When you think of it, they live completely on the charity of their family, never have a shilling of their own to buy a bar of chocolate or even a penny to give to a child. Do you think that it would be possible to work out a scheme to give people like that, without any entitlement to anything, a few bob a week of their own?' I asked him if he wanted me to tackle it, and he said to 'go ahead', and I did. It was really an adminsitrative affair but there was a large medical content to it. So I blocked out a scheme and Tom Murphy organised the County Medical Officers to use their district nurses to seek out such people. They then assessed them and determined their entitlements and in a very short time we had the Disabled Persons Allowances Scheme. It did not cost a lot but was a boon to thousands of poor people who were disabled for life, like my friend the little man at the side of the road. It may sound a bit corny, but that's how it happened and it was due to an impulse on the part of James Ryan.

I told Dr Ryan about our adventures in setting up the quarantine room in the Legion of Mary Hostel and about the place generally and one day he said that he would like to see it. After a bit of trouble getting them to let us in, we walked about looking at everything and as Dr Ryan said nothing, one could see Frank Duff growing increasingly uneasy and wondering what we were up to and fearful lest we might close the place down. The place was pretty grim. It had been the old workhouse for North Dublin, and had been battered about in 1916. It had been handed to the Legion in a semi-derelict state, and they used it among other things as a hostel for unmarried mothers and their babies. Here and there, through those great empty workhouse wards, the women had made little private areas. An old bed, a cradle made from an orange-box, a couple of other such boxes for a bedside table or a stool, a rag of a floor rug, pin-ups and holy pictures and a clothes line and this was their home. The women went out to work as cleaners and such like and the children were cared-for. As they grew up, Frank saw to their schooling and eventually found them jobs or apprenticed them to trades. Just before leaving, Dr Ryan turned suddenly and said, 'Frank, I'll give you £30,000 Sweep money, give each woman a decent cubicle, fix up the sanitation and the heating and so on, and when you have finished, let me know and I will come and see it.' Frank nearly fainted with joy. He got so excited that he turned off his hearing aid and did not know what he was saying or whether he was coming or going. That was James Ryan, a delightful able gentleman with a good heart. It was a pleasure to work for him.

The third Minister, and the most unusual, was Noel Browne. He was in the chair for three years, from 1948 to 1951. In one sense he was simply an episode in a series of ministers who were the political heads of the Department, while we, the medical team, pursued and organised a new health service and so on, but in another he was more than a mere episode and his reign had a major effect on my life.

I first met him in 1945, so far as I can remember. I had a friend called Kennedy, whom I knew in Queen's. He wrote to me and said that he was a patient in Newcastle Sanatorium, Co Wicklow and would like me to come to see him if I could. Now Newcastle was an unusual place in that although small, it had a Medical Superintendent, with Browne as assistant MO, and a visiting staff of 'distinguished' Dublin consultants who came to visit, do rounds and prescribe treatment. These consultants must have been hard to take for Browne, who had been trained in top English sanatoria, had been ill himself and understood the disease and was doing most of the work on a small salary. The Newcastle Sanatorium was a small, voluntary place, had little funds, some of the patients paid for their keep and the consultant's services and the hospital had changed little in the fifty years of its existence. After sitting at my desk all week, exercise was necessary, so from time to time I cycled down to see Harry Kennedy either in

Newcastle or later in Kilmacanogue where he had a house. These Sunday cycle rides were pleasant and I enjoyed his company. He introduced me to Noel Browne and indeed said that Browne had put him up to writing to me. Kennedy was a very clever man and a brilliant journalist but because of his illness and because he was doing badly had become very frustrated. Browne and Kennedy were two very 'angry young men'.

Both Kennedy and Browne were very critical and indeed scournful of the way Newcastle Sanatorium, and the service generally, were run. It was no use telling them that I had things moving, that I was just as angry and concerned as they were and that we were going ahead just as fast as was possible. I believed that there was more to ending TB than sanatoria and the treatment of patients with the disease.

At that time, I found Browne a very interesting character. He had been very ill with tuberculosis himself and was lucky to be alive. Because of this, and other reasons which at the time I did not know, he was very kind indeed to the patients, who adored him. Most of his professional life had been spent in TB institutions of one form or other, large or small, here or in England. Now, just as patients can become institutionalised, so can staff, and life for such staff people becomes a matter of living in a small world, with limited human experience and equally limited medical experience. Even if poorly paid, they had tenure, security, things like houses provided and sometimes other amenities such as laundry, heating and maid attendance. They were generally well taken care of. Browne certainly was influenced by this institutional experience as regards his medical outlook but equally he identified with the patients in Newcastle and they appreciated him. He was undoubtedly a very clever man, with a strange background which made him interesting. He had gone as far as he could go in Newcastle and was about ready to burst out somewhere, some place or in some way. At the same time, he was intolerant, begrudging of other's efforts and, while a magnificent destructive critic, which at that time was easy, he had few constructive or practical ideas. However he was likeable, certainly compassionate and had a lot going for him.

Sometime towards the end of 1947, I was rung up in the Custom House by someone speaking for Superintendents of

Sanatoria, who had formed an advisory group and who asked
if they might come to see me and advise on TB. I made them
welcome. I had already had discussions with the County
Medical Officers and with some of the consultants on the
Dublin teaching hospitals such as Dr Eddie Freeman, who was
a good friend of mine, so I was ready to meet them. The TB
scheme was going well and we had the building plans for the
regional sanatoria drafted and ready to go ahead. Also we
were about to issue a White Paper on the Programme. When
on the Rockefeller Fellowship, I had made friends with some
of the Canadian tuberculosis people and found that their
sanatoria were very good and they had promised me to take
some of our doctors for study/training jobs if we sent them
over. I wanted to discuss the selection of the people to send
with these superintendents.

The group came in, with Noel Browne as Secretary; I outlined the scheme to them and made a general presentation on
the subject and produced the plans of the sanatoria for their
criticism and advice. The discussion proceeded pleasantly until
Browne took over. He made a lot of scathing remarks and was
downright rude and insolent. Now I had stuck my neck out
on this thing, had taken it in hand, got it going and was producing results. So, I was not about to take calculated rudeness
from a young sanatorium assistant, no matter how able, whose
experience was extremely limited and whose remarks anyway
were not helpful. Since he continued and no one could stop
him, I terminated the meeting.

At that time, there was a continuous barrage of criticism
from people who had never done anything but who were
remarkably good at talking. The ending of tuberculosis was a
technical thing, but they used it as a very handy political
weapon with which to beat the government.

The next day, someone from the group rang again on their
behalf, apologised and asked might they return and I said
'yes, but without Browne'. I saw them again, they came in as
often as they wished and our relations were pleasant and their
advice valuable. The day after, Browne rang and asked might
he come in. I said to come along and he did and apologised
for his remarks. We discussed things in a completely friendly
way. In the conversation, he said that he appreciated what I

had managed to do so far and asked whether I would have any objection to his raising the matter of TB in public outside of medical circles. I said certainly not, the more well-informed pressure outside, the better chance we had 'inside', of pushing things on. He talked about political pressure and I said that I could not advise him. We parted on what I thought were friendly terms.

Without my knowing it, this visit more or less coincided with the foundation of the Clann na Poblachta party of which Browne was a member. This party had as one of its main party planks a violent criticism of the handling of the tuberculosis problem by the Fianna Fáil government. It seemed to me that this was largely inspired by Browne.

In December 1947 I published a study I had done some time before of the tuberculosis deaths in Lurgan which had occurred in the town over a period of twenty-five years. It showed that this was a slow-moving contagious disease. When the deaths were plotted on maps of working class streets and the time factor was taken into account, they could be seen to occur in 'clusters'. There were in fact small slow-moving localised epidemics. They started from one focus, flared up over a period of years and then burnt out.

The next month the paper was attacked in two separate letters to the *Journal of the Irish Medical Association* by Dr Browne and a Dr Galvin from England. Dr Galvin made a reasonable criticism that the results could have been random and therefore invalid. Roy Geary, whom I had consulted on the statistics of the paper, got very mad at this attack and did an independent study and proved that I was right. Professor Eddie Conway, the Professor of Biochemistry in UCD, and the father of bio-chemical micro-analysis, the greatest research man we have produced in medicine in this century, also confirmed my analysis. The Oxford School of Social Medicine carried out the same kind of study in Northampton, after mine, and found the same result. It became known elsewhere and MacDougall, the Chief of Tuberculosis in the World Health Organisation, wrote it up in the Italian *Tuberculosis Journal* and said 'I have given special consideration to this study by Deeny because it is a searching attempt to trace tuberculosis disease to its source, and is an example of the type of survey which might well be repeated in many towns and villages in many countries'.

Browne's attack on the other hand was unreasonable and more. It was impolite, personal and really political. Within a week or two of its publication however, as a result of the success of Clann na Poblachta in the elections of February 1948, Dr Browne was appointed Minister of Health and my chief. The amusement in medical circles in Dublin at this situation was very great. I was rung up by two Fine Gael ministers in the government and asked would I work with Browne. One was Dr Tom O'Higgins and the other James Dillon, with whom I had been at school and who was a friend. I answered both the same way. 'We have this whole programme well in hand and nothing must stop it. If they sent along Satan himself I would work with him to end TB and to save babies lives.'

The next day, we had a meeting of the medical staff and we discussed the whole thing. I was very much on edge since I did not know what this new man would do to the work that we had spent years in bringing to the point we had reached. Others were concerned as well as me. Theo MacWeeney expected trouble, as did J.D. MacCormack. Charles Lysaght was unhappy at any threat to the hospital building programme we had drawn up. We were all uneasy. In the end we decided that according to our civil service tradition and in the interest of the people we served that we should give him our total support, without reservation. We took ourselves very seriously then, because at the back of our minds always was the spectre of lost lives.

When Browne arrived in his office as Minister, I went to see him and welcomed him on behalf of the medical staff. He referred to the comments he had made on my paper on tuberculosis, and I said that I had written a reply and he said that I should go ahead and publish it. This was now impossible; I would have to be content that he would read it. He said he would, so I gave him the manuscript. I filled him in on what we had done recently in respect of TB and what was in progress, for example the 2,000 beds which we had earmarked and were in process of taking over, staffing, equipping and filling with patients. To my surprise, he was quite unaware of the situation. He was assured of the support of the medical staff and he thanked me. The next day or so, he went public and announced that he had found it possible to produce 2,000 extra tuberculosis beds.

For the next few months, things went well and everyone was happy. Different developments that we had planned and organised came about and he got the credit. His star was in the ascendant. There was no doubt but at this time his appointment was working satisfactorily. The TB patients were delighted, since he was very popular with them. The young people throughout the country thought that he was wonderful, as indeed he was. He also had complete medical support at this time. He seemed to be patently sincere, had great energy, was an attractive personality and had a great deal going for him. After all the 'stick' that the Department had had from the press, to receive praise for the good works of the Minister was wonderful. He had two great speech writers and advisers on media matters in Aodh de Blacam and Frank Galagher. Being a politician and as was reasonable and to be expected, he exploited this situation very successfully. As he came from the relatively closed world of a small sanatorium, the medical staff and I spent quite a lot of time with him trying to sense him into the national medical scene, its problems and what we were doing about them.

However after about a year, from our point of view things started to go wrong. Ministers when appointed often have ideas of what they want to do or commitments to either party or friends or to pressure groups. Sean MacBride, in an interview, stated that Dr Browne apparently intended to control the medical profession by building up the Trinity influence against UCD or some such ploy. The interesting but frustrating division between UCD, the Royal Colleges and TCD was a relic of the development of medical education. For many generations TCD had been the ascendancy school and so supreme. Then in the middle of the last century a challenge came from the Catholics and gradually a Catholic Medical School emerged. This developed into the National University with University College Dublin in combat with Trinity. The Royal Colleges of Physicians and Surgeons also gradually asserted their independence. At times the situation was difficult and bitter and there were of course clerical and political implications. So far as health planning was concerned, the jealousy between the schools meant that they would rarely agree. There were other matters. For example Browne wanted to build a cancer hospital. Since Dublin had already two small cancer hospitals I felt that we did not need a third. I was also against small specialist hospitals and believed that any cancer development should be part of a large general hospital such as the new St Vincent's which we had already activated and which would deal with a lot of cancer anyway. Or we could enlarge the existing Northbrook Road Cancer Hospital. The new hospital as proposed was to be on the lines of the Holt/Christie in Manchester, which I had seen, appreciated very much in one sense, but did not like since it was almost confined to radio-therapy and in my view was too restricted to this form of treatment. There is a lot more to cancer than radio-therapy. The hospital was the brain-child of Dr Oliver Chance. He became its first director. But the go-ahead was given to create St Luke's. Now to be fair, St Luke's has given an excellent service throughout the years since and thousands of people have been treated there and we have no way of knowing what would have happened had we chosen another line. Later on, I became a member of the Board of Governors and tried to coordinate the work between the three hospitals, but still feel that it was a mistake to have built it.

Another project Dr Browne took up was the building of a new fever hospital at Cherry Orchard. This had been on the planning board for years. It was all mixed up with politics, since it had been the focus of a bitter political battle a few years before. We had already two fever hospitals in Dublin, largely empty even though one was a bit decrepit. Gurranebraher Hospital in Cork had been built as a fever place before the war, but had never been opened. But typhoid, typhus and diphtheria were on their way out, the streptococcus had lost its virulence and things like scarletina and all the acute rheumatic fevers were on the wane. The two existing institutions were quite adequate for the moment until we could see where things were going. I have a memory of writing across the front of the main file, 'the building of this hospital is quite unnecessary'. But the order was given to build Cherry Orchard Fever

Hospital at the cost, in today's figures, of a great many millions. The new Cherry Orchard Fever Hospital has looked after very many thousands of patients, and in the 'polio' days it was a great centre. Under Harry O'Flanagan's guidance and with the cooperation of the excellent staff it became, after Copenhagen, one of the most advanced places for the care of bulbar 'polio' anywhere.

There was the matter of BCG. We had a scheme started in Dublin and going well, and which as a further development we wanted to extend to the rest of the country as part of the TB service under the Chief Medical Officers of counties. The basic idea was to integrate it into the tuberculosis service. This was side-tracked and a National BCG Committee, influenced by Dorothy Price and based on St Ultan's Hospital was set up to operate a National BCG campaign, which would cooperate with the CMOs but would remain a separate entity. The first Director was Dr Cowell. Our objection was that we had enough of these independent groups floating around, each doing their own thing; for this job we wanted a close-knit integrated organisation. Also, I was horrified at the idea of placing it in St Ultan's which was already a hospital for advanced tuberculous children and where there was always a risk of cross-infection and contamination of the BCG vaccine, no matter how careful you were. However, to be fair, Dr Cowell did an excellent job and deserves the greatest credit for his achievement not only in the vaccination of vast numbers of children but for the close and happy relationship he maintained with the CMOs.

New faces, in addition to the Trinity people, began to appear in the Custom House, whether as advisers or PROs or people given minor posts, but who represented for example, post-sanatorium patients and who, through Dick White, his private secretary, an ex post office detective, had access to the Minister, a sort of mafia which had not been seen before in the Irish civil service. The medical staff saw Dr Browne less and less, and there was a sense of unease about the place. We might well have been worried, since he had invited in an advisory committee to prepare a Mother and Child Scheme. This to say the least was odd, since my colleagues and I had been working on it for some years and it had been ready to go since

1947. It seems foolish not to have asked us about it, particularly since it was I who thought it up and planned it in the first instance. Anyway, what they came up with was very little different from what I prepared in 1946.

About this time Dr Gerry O'Brien of the Richmond Hospital, who had been in Clongowes with me and who was a life-long friend of mine, was President of the student's Scientific Society of the Royal College of Surgeons. He was due to give his Presidential address and asked me to speak to the paper. I said, 'Ask our new young Minister, it'll be good for him to meet the students and he likes all the publicity that he can get. If he does not do it, I will.' The Minister accepted Gerry's invitation and he was sent a copy of the address. It was quite harmless, and not controversial, since it praised some unknown medical heroes of Ireland. Dr Browne asked me to write his speech for him and I did; it agreed that these men were indeed heroes and that we needed more people like them today and some such other sentiments. It was a nice dignified ministerial statement.

I did not go to hear him, but that evening and the next morning, I was rung up by various people and asked 'Has he gone nuts?' They told me that everything had been peaceable and going along nicely when suddenly the Minister folded up his paper, put it in his pocket and launched into a fairly violent attack on the doctors. He had barely resumed his seat, when Leonard Abrahamson, Bob Collis and a string of other senior people who were there replied just as viciously and vehemently. The consultants' exasperation was fuelled by the extensive use of Sweep monies for the regional hospital programme, rather than for the Dublin voluntary hospitals the original desination, many of which had substantial deficits. They were also galled by the Minister's use of a student occasion to raise these issues. I was so upset that later the next morning I asked to see him.

I asked him why, when the Minister of Justice did not attack the Gardaí or the lawyers, or the Minister of Agriculture the farmers, Ministers of Health always seemed to want to bash the doctors. They were no better or no worse than any other group and since we could not do without their goodwill, we had been cultivating good relations with them for years. I felt that he was wrong in what he had done and should try to repair the damage. I also told him that Dr Ward had been aggressive and in consequence had a tough time with his health bill, while James Ryan took things easily and had little medical opposition to the 1947 Act. My reception was not cordial. Up till then Dr Browne had the general support of the Irish doctors, he threw it away and for his own reasons antagonised them.

From that point on, things became very difficult. We saw him less and less. He developed a little court of administrative people. This included the architects, who went through the ritual of keeping tabs on the building progress and so on. I was told that things were as bad for some of the senior administrators as for me.

It was also quite impossible to satisfy him on how inspections were carried out. For example, I would be sent for, and told to carry out an inspection into some affair in a Dublin sanatorium. This would be in front of the 'Court', and so staged as possibly to humiliate me. When I returned to my room, I would find that the file I had been handed contained the complaint from someone, enclosed in a sealed envelope which was not to be opened. This kind of thing was all wrong, and became rather difficult when you went out and found nothing.

The 'hassle' over the inspections got so bad that I had to draw up 'standing orders' with which an inspector had to comply, with signed statements and witnessed signatures from every one concerned and check-lists and so on, like a police enquiry only without the fingerprinting. All this to try to obviate bias or prejudice in favour of staffs as against the patients and of course a political stunt. In the end the place from my point of view became paranoidal.

I had started a survey of dispensaries under James Ryan, as I have already explained, and this kept the younger men out and busy and away from all this nonsense. From time to time, Browne would send one of his coterie to ask me was it finished? I understand that he referred to it as something significant in submissions to the government. Mr MacGilligan, the Minister of Finance turned him down about something in a letter of March 1951 because of this redistribution of dispensaries.

At times I felt that Browne was ruthless and much more calculating than people thought and indeed possibly vindictive. One day I got a note instructing me to take Theo MacWeeney off TB. Just like that, no reason given. I pointed out that Theo knew more about TB than anyone else in Ireland and that with a TB campaign on, it was shortsighted to take him off TB. He then said that Theo could deal with TB files, but was not to carry out any inspections or be seen to have anything to do with it. Theo anguished around the place for a while, and it was hard to see his distress as he had worked harder than anyone for years on TB. He felt that it was his life's work. We were equally upset but could do nothing.

Theo applied to WHO for a job and they took him on immediately since people like him were hard to find in the TB world. They made him Regional Adviser on TB to the governments of the eight countries of South East Asia with a population of more than one billion people. He had a great success and was beloved all over Asia and was retained as a Consultant by WHO, at the request of governments, for years after he had retired. But he was not good enough for Browne.

One of the problems concerning Browne was that most of his administrators were new to the field of health development work. They had come in a couple of years before and although highly intelligent capable people as civil service officers, had never encountered a situation such as this and could exercise little influence over him.

The worsening situation in the Custom House got me down. I could not sleep because of it and wandered up and down outside my house in Portmarnock early in the morning or half of the night. I was worrying that what we had worked so hard to achieve was being smashed up. Looking back on it, it all seems so silly now, but there was real anguish at the time, particularly when he pulled stunts like going on the radio and inviting anyone with a complaint against a doctor to approach him.

The whole thing gradually became public. One day John Shiels, a solicitor and a friend of my father, whom I knew to be prominent in the Knights of St Columbanus, stopped me in the street and said, 'I hear that you are in trouble. Don't worry, nothing will happen to you,' and passed on. Another day, Jack Saunders, the CMO for Cork City and at that time the President of the Society of Medical Officers of Health came up from Cork and offered me the support of the Society to do anything I felt necessary and discussed the question of what to do with the way things were going. This offered comfort, but there was nothing they could do. The medical people in the Department were as helpless as I was while I waited my turn for the 'chop'.

I was so fed up with the nonsense that I considered getting out and starting to practice somewhere outside Dublin. After all I could always earn a living and believed that in a year or two in practice anywhere, I could earn more than I was getting in the Custom House as Chief Medical Adviser. I had been a good practitioner and I could become one again. I remember going down to Limerick to look at houses with a view to going there to practise. Finally, it became obvious the whole thing was a comedy; the situation could not last, so I decided to hang on and be available to help to pick up the pieces when things changed.

I need not have worried quite so much, since he left Charlie Lysaght alone and did not interfere very much with the hospital building programme which we had restarted after the war and which was based on the 1945 Plan. This had been accepted even by Browne himself, and was still being implemented by him as by his predecessors as though it had been approved and not turned down by the 1945 Cabinet. As I said earlier, no one had looked at the dispensary service for a hundred years and we wanted proposals to consider how to bring it up to date. So I made myself busy with this while I was isolated.

Dr Browne had a penchant for publicity in all ways, great and small. One of his minor efforts was to offer a £50 prize for a slogan promoting the national tuberculosis effort. In 1948 £50 was a lot of money. I was walking along one of the corridors in the Custom House one morning and just as I passed his office, Myles na gCopaleen came out and in a furtive conspiratorial manner, stopped me and said 'I have been looking for you to tell you that I have just won the slogan competition'. 'Good,' says I, 'what's your slogan?' He put his finger to his nose and whispered 'TB's bad for you!' and popped back into his office like a ferret down a rabbit burrow.

When the 'chop' came it was like this. Quite unexpectedly, Mr O'Cinneide, the Secretary, sent for me one day, and after a few minutes of polite chit-chat asked me casually whether I would consider being seconded out for a while to take over St James's Hospital, the huge old municipal institution. My job would be to turn it into a first-class hospital. In civil service terms this was as near as the Minister could go to dismissal. I asked the Secretary 'what about a budget?' 'You will have all that you might need to do a good job,' he said. I came back later and asked 'would I have administrative authority?' and he said 'no!'. So I turned it down. The administrative commissioner was a very fine old gentleman called Seaumas Murphy, who regarded the place as his own hospital and he was not going to like any intruder such as me. Equally I could not do a job with Seaumas breathing down the back of my neck and trying to control everything.

For some time before this I had been planning a National Tuberculosis Survey, which I had hoped would be carried out by Theo MacWeeney. There were a lot of questions to be answered. We needed to define very clearly our problem, to secure much more information on the factors favouring the spread of the disease and as we were improving and extending our organisation we needed to know how best to do it. We also needed to work out a lot of new techniques applicable to Ireland. This would have gone ahead earlier had it not been for the nonsense in the Department.

After Theo's departure to WHO, I put it up to the Secretary that if seconded out to the Medical Research Council, I would do the job myself. The proposal was accepted immediately and I was free. Not once, before I left, did Dr Browne discuss the project with me, nor during the Survey did he once visit us to see what we were doing or ask for a progress report. He had got rid of me, and from then on he was not only Minister, but his own Chief Medical Adviser and TB expert and that was that.

The Medical Research Council agreed to accept responsibility for the Survey. UCD had just acquired Montrose, the present RTE centre, as part of the plan for the acquisition of lands for the new Belfield campus. They had it available at the time and I was lucky since they gave it to me for the head-quarters of the Survey. I moved into the large empty house, with a table and a couple of chairs and I was in business. The survey took three years, which meant that I was out of the Department during the heat of the Mother and Child contro-versy. I became so preoccupied with the Survey, that I paid little attention to it.

Ever since 1950-51, the 'Mother and Child' row has been a matter of intense public interest and this has lasted for more than thirty-five years. Thinking and writing about the Mother and Child has a fascination for me now, partly because I was the one to dream up the scheme and to name it. During the ten years while people messed about with it and before I could see it in action the most incredible things happened to it; bloody-mindedness, bad luck, folly, idiocy, scheming, religious obscurancy, politics, government crises, defeats, anxieties, ideologies, all over the simple matter of introducing a simple scheme, which we needed and could afford, to save children's lives and enable them to grow up in a healthy fashion.

In Ireland, during the period from 1930 to 1950, the Catholic Church had reached its peak of power, prosperity and effective organisation. There was an abundance of vocations and a very large number of clerics held key positions of great power. Yet the growth in State power disturbed them. There were signs that this was increasing and would increase. They were worried that the Family was threatened, that the old way of rural and small town life was changing and that somehow this was not good.

The Papal Encyclical *Rerum Novarum* published in 1891 laid down Catholic teaching on the duty of Society to the Worker and the duty of the Worker to Society. It was brought up to date in 1931 by a further Encyclical *Quadregesimo Anno*. These, coupled with their anxiety on social conditions, led the clergy to advocate a Corporate or Vocational society. They had great opportunities to pursue this. The Bishop of Galway, Michael Browne, was Chairman of the Vocational Commission. The Bishop of Clonfert, Dr Dignan, was Chair-man of the National Health Insurance Society. Father Eddie Coyne S.J. was Chairman of the Irish Agricultural Wholesale Society, which controlled the Cooperative Movement. Father

Hayes of Tipperary, the founder of Muintir na Tir, had enormous influence with rural people. The Jesuits had a College
of Industrial Relations where they trained trades union personnel. The leading hospitals were managed by religious orders
as were almost all secondary schools and the clergy held a
large number of important university chairs. They had taught
all the leading people in government, in the professions and
virtually everyone had a relation a priest or a nun, so that they
were enmeshed in the social fabric in every community. They
were on good terms with most people and they tried to sell
the corporate idea as something which this State should adopt.

I know about this because I started my indoctrination at
fourteen years of age as a member of the Social Study Club
in Clongowes in 1920 and thereafter was pretty well mixed
up with it for years. They did not go about it as a kind of
Rome Rule conspiracy, but if you add up all the different
manifestations as J.H. Whyte does in his book *Church and
State in Modern Ireland*, a pattern can be seen. What they
wanted was a plural society. Not a pluralist society as we en-
visage to-day accommodating all shades of ethical and religious
views, but a society of plural institutions. It was not a question
of Rome rule, but of a responsible society, with a maximum
amount of decentralisation, local community groups, industries and professions remaining independent and the preser-
vation of the family as the basic unit of society. The law of
subsidiarity should exist in that a senior, centralised instrument
of government should not undertake tasks which could be
performed equally well by a junior agent. The clergy were
highly motivated since they were clearly aware of the serious
social conditions and poverty. Archbishop MacQuaid of Dublin
had established the Catholic Social Service Conference: among
other things it provided more than two million free meals each
year for the Dublin poor. There was also a remarkable crop
of extraordinary people around such as Frank Duff, who
founded the Legion of Mary, an international organisation
with millions of members all over the world and active in
almost a thousand Catholic dioceses mainly in the Third World.
Mother Mary Martin, who founded the Medical Missionaries
of Mary, built a new hospital for her doctors and nurses every
year for thirty years. There was the Irish spiritual empire of

thousands of missionaries all over the Third World.

Forty years on, it is difficult to appreciate the strength of this movement but one can still see its effects. It influenced Mr de Valera in his design for the Senate under his Constitution. This was conceived along vocational lines. However it produced a reaction, in that people felt that the all-encompassing influence might become something of a theocracy. They became afraid of it. And then the clergy over-played their hand. They over-played their hand by moving away from doing what they had done so successfully, educating and promoting a responsible caring society of a plurality of institutions. They blindly accepted the notion of a confrontation, which in hindsight was unnecessary folly.

One of the key ingredients in the brew was an extraordinary but sincere and dedicated man called James MacPolin, Chief Medical Officer for Limerick, who had composed a theology based on St Thomas Aquinas, Maritain and other modern French Christian philosophers, with bits from Kant and from Hegel, adding a masterly interpretation of the Papal Encyclicals. He preached this theology as a theme against bureaucracy, totalitarianism, modernism, the use of modern science, and against what he considered were scientific fascists like me, who were perverting the moral basis of society by the exercise and exploitation of political power. Despite his official position as CMO for Limerick, he took on this crusade more or less as a whole time job and developed a power base or following among the local medical people in the city and county. In the Department we became worried about the situation. MacPolin was here and there and everywhere, making speeches to small groups and societies and on one occasion Des Hourihan and I went down to Limerick to talk to him. On another occasion, when James Ryan went to address the Limerick Council, just before the 1947 Health Act was passed, he took me with him for support. All went well, till MacPolin got up and denounced me, amongst other things for invading the pages of the medical journals with Departmental propaganda. James Ryan defended me, and the meeting became devoted to the right of the Chief Medical Adviser to publish research papers in medical journals, with all the local councillors joining in.

In the *Journal of the Medical Association of Ireland* for

August of 1946, I had published the account of my typhoid study and the strategy for ending the disease in this country. In the same Journal MacPolin published a monograph embodying his thesis. It was in two parts in the August and September issues, the whole of about 15,000 words. He called this 'Aspects of the Sociology of the Medical Profession'. It is very closely written and hard to read, but in it he outlines not really the sociology but the theology of state medicine. He describes it as interfering with the privacy of the family, as derogating from the responsibility of parents for their children, of the role and authority of parents, of the family as a sacred unit and so on and so on. In it he defies the state and claims the right to speak as he likes. This provided the thesis, blueprint, scenario, or rationale or whatever for one side of the Mother and Child controversy.

He sold it over a period to the Irish Medical Association, although I believe that a large section of the profession never really understood what he was talking about. Then with the profession's backing he sold it to the bishops. Now, it was written in semi-theological language which the bishops understood and gave them the basis for their stand and in fact their confrontation with the state. Thenceforth anything James MacPolin might say was likely to be acceptable to the bishops. He had two uncles who were parish priests, one being Dean of Dromore. He had a sister a nun in Lurgan and of course there was Monsignor Eugene the wonderful Founder of the Maynooth Mission to China, so they were likely to trust him, especially since he spoke their language.

The ultimate confrontation was folly on the part of the bishops. There was no need for it. It alienated a great number of people, destroyed relationships and brought about the opposition of politicians, bureaucrats, intellectuals and indeed the people who plainly saw the need for a public health programme for children. They had chosen or allowed themselves to be persuaded to fight on the wrong issue.

In doing so, tragically they came up against a minister, Dr Noel Browne, who had insufficient negotiating experience, not enough knowledge of the subject matter of Maternity and Child Welfare, without guidance or restraint from Cabinet, Party or Leader, all of whom he seems to have alienated, and depending on a medical profession whom he had antagonized. When one examines this side of the story, it is incredible. The process of change in public health matters was in progress but it was obviously a difficult, even explosive situation which required very careful handling by experienced politicians and statesmen. In dealing with legislation, dialogue and negotiation then compromise, good sense and at the same time, firmness were required. At stake were the lives of thousands. Therefore the introduction of Dr Browne to the Department was unfortunate, and difficult to understand, for various reasons.

Firstly, the government, while fully aware of this situation, appointed Browne, a quite inexperienced young man, no matter how able, as Minister, and expected him, without political guidance or restraint, to deal with a major controversial programme.

Secondly, the government, purely on a basis of political expediency in awarding a minority party in coalition a ministerial post, allowed him free rein to do as he liked and then, when the 'crunch' came, withdrew support immediately and reneged on their stated policy.

Thirdly, the government, again on a basis of political expediency, appointed someone whom Mr Costello, the Taoiseach, would later describe as 'not competent or capable to fulfil the duties of the Department of Health' and about whom Sean MacBride, the leader of Dr Browne's party, would say 'For the last year, in my view the Minister of Health has not been normal'.

So a foolish and unnecessary confrontation occurred between the Bishops, inspired by James MacPolin and backed by the doctors, and this most unusual and somewhat extraordinary young man. A Minister who became isolated and alienated from his cabinet and party which promptly disowned the policy which they had previously adopted. This destroyed him and indeed the government itself and caused a church-state crisis which had a profound effect on the country. Between the lot of them they made a right mess of the Mother and Child scheme. The real tragedy of the debacle was that it set back public health in the country for years and opened up the way to the centralised, bureaucratic, politicised and authoritarian government which we now enjoy.

8

The National Tuberculosis Survey 1950-53

I N 1851, Sir William Willis O'Flaherty Wilde, Oscar's father, was made a Commissioner of the second Census carried out in this country. He had been a consultant for the first in 1841. He carried out not only the Census but also the first Comprehensive National Morbidity Study, in fact a national census of deaths and diseases, the first in any country ever.

He arranged that the police when they called to take the census to each house in the country would ask if anyone was sick and ascertain what was wrong with them. They were also asked if there had been any deaths in the house during the previous ten years, and if so, what were the causes.

The work in Dublin was done in greater detail. Wilde related the deaths to age, sex, occupation and residence. For example he divided the city into first, second and third-class shop streets. The same for residential streets and the rest were included in the Liberties of the Archbishop of Dublin, or the Liberties of the Earl of Meath. It is a fascinating glimpse into the past.

As regards tuberculosis, there were first-class trades people like carvers and gilders, printers and workers in gold and silver who had only a slight mortality from the disease. But it was clear that TB was related to living conditions: of 194 deaths of servants in houses in first-class residential streets, 31 (16%) were due to consumption; of 370 deaths of persons living in second-class streets, 108 (29%) were due to consumption; and of 926 deaths of servants living in third-class residential streets, 321 (35%) were due to consumption, showing a steady increase in the rate with diminishing social status.

When you consider that this survey was carried out under the wretched post-famine conditions, by policemen going on foot from house to house, analysed and written up by clerks writing in long-hand, it was an extraordinary feat. The final reports were beautifully produced, the tables were engraved and the volumes bound in leather.

Medical circles in Dublin have more or less canonised Stokes, Colles, Adams, Corrigan and the rest of the Victorian 'greats', but there was none as good as old Wilde. He was the first anthropologist in this country and his skull collection was unique. He wrote beautifully and his description of the nature and beauty of the great rivers of Ireland and the country-side are superb. He was probably the first person ever to have seen the living ear-drum, because he invented the auriscope. 'Wilde's Incision' for the operation of mastoidectomy must have saved the lives of thousands and thousands of people each year for a hundred years and more. He founded a hospital and was a great Gaelic scholar. Unfortunately he did not wash a lot, was an ugly little man and blotted his copy-book with a lady (or rather she blotted it for him) but these were small faults in a great scientist.

There was no name to the report which the Local Government submitted to the International Tuberculosis Conference in Washington in 1908. I believe it was written by Sir Thomas Stafford-King-Harman, a worthy baronet, who had started off as Tommy Stafford, a dispensary doctor in Jamestown, but who, with the appropriate embellishments, ended up in a job more or less the same as mine. The report stated 'As malnutrition, bad housing and sanitation and all other circumstances of poverty were with us even in a more pronounced form, long before the increase in the tubercular death-rate, it cannot, we think, be deduced from the facts before us that they have been the cause of the excessive death rate from tuberculosis'. The report went on to give what were believed to be the true reasons:

1) The domestic or home treatment of advanced cases of tuberculosis;
2) Ignorance of the true nature of the disease and the proper methods to prevent or limit infection.

It was clear that the provision of sufficient sanatorium beds to isolate cases from their families would be sufficient to take care of 'the domestic or home treatment of advanced cases of Tuberculosis', so that the home nursing of tuberculosis was unnecessary. But to conquer the disease we needed to find out as much as possible about it and how to formulate the most effective methods to prevent or limit infection.

This is what I proposed to do through the National Tuberculosis Survey.

The history of the disease in Ireland showed that the great national epidemic began in the two decades before the Famine years. Judging from the bones found in archaeological digs, there was no bone TB in Ireland 1,000 years ago. Looking at Bills of Mortality for Dublin, starting in 1661, it was interesting to see the role of parish clerks as registrars and particularly of 'searchers' who were old women who visited houses where deaths had occurred and ascertained the cause of death. The disease then seems to have been largely confined to towns, particularly Dublin. It increased in intensity during the second half of the nineteenth century. Apart from small remissions it reached its peak at the beginning of the twentieth century and since then has abated. The reduction in deaths, which was interrupted during the two world wars, was slowed down in the period by population changes, principally urbanisation. This reduction had increased with dramatic rapidity within the last few years.

Now in scientific work, one has to be properly humble. Wise old men may not have the answer but they can point the way. The idea of a survey, which had been simmering in my mind for a long time, undoubtedly came from turning over and thinking about the things these old men said or did and linking their ideas to modern concepts and problems.

One of the approaches we were to use in the survey was that of the newly-emerging discipline of ecology. This is the science of plants and animals in relation to their environment. A doctor faced with a case of tuberculosis was exercised mainly on how he should cure the patient. Politicians, administrators and the public faced with cases sought to isolate them in sanatoria and treat them, hopefully to effect a cure. I preferred to regard the tubercle bacillus as a parasite having an existence or ecology of its own and for its survival:

1) The parasite must gain entrance to the host — man,

2) It must adapt and multiply inside the host, usually in the lungs,

3) There must be an exit from the host by migration or discharge,

4) There must be an effective mechanism for transmission to a new host. In this way it causes the disease.

This concept was originated by Theobald Smith in Princeton in 1934 and then promulgated by Thomas Francis and René Dubos in America. It was never sufficiently considered or adopted on this side of the Atlantic.

As regards the Survey, my interest in ecology was two-fold. Firstly, how the tubercle bacillus existed in the Irish community, how it maintained itself, how it spread from one human to another, what were the factors favouring its spread and, in particular, how to interrupt the spread of transmission. In effect, we were to study the relationship of the tubercle bacillus as a parasite to its human host and environment.

Secondly, we wanted to define the problem in Ireland exactly and also to find out why the bacillus should invade one person, and cause breakdown of lung tissue, and not another person. What factors favoured the invasion? What had things like age, occupation, sex, domicile and other such features got to do with the spread of infection? What happened when the human was invaded? How did the tissues react? How could we identify people who had been invaded? Then we needed to define a national strategy to eradicate the disease. I made my request to be allowed out to do the Survey towards the end of May 1950 and by August, I had Montrose and had started to work.

I decided to approach the thing on three main fronts. First, a survey and definition of the natural problem involving deaths, cases, factors favouring spread and the development of techniques, with special emphasis of radiology. Second, a study of the ecology of the tubercle bacillus itself. Third, the statistical evaluation of the problem, based on the material collected by the Survey and an assessment of the findings. This meant staff, radiological equipment, a laboratory and a battery of statistical machinery.

We began by studying the deaths from the disease which

had taken place in the twelve years between 1938 and 1949. These numbered 43,007. They were fairly evenly divided between the sexes with slightly more males dying than females. There was proportionately a larger number and higher rate in Dublin than elsewhere in the country. More males died in Dublin than females and the reverse was seen down the country. More young females died and 56 per cent of all female deaths were in the age groups of 15 to 35 years. More males died amongst the older age groups and 49 per cent of all males dying were over 35. The main finding was the large proportion of male and female pulmonary tuberculosis deaths occurring in early adult life. There was a great amount of detailed information coming from this part of the survey and we were beginning to see a picture or pattern emerge. The tragedy of 43,007 preventable deaths, mainly of young people, was a sobering thought.

Then we did a Morbidity Study. This was of immense interest since we were now getting down to live cases. It was of added importance since it represented more or less an evaluation of the services we had provided up to this. In Ireland, each county or county borough had a tuberculosis register (a list of all reported) which included all the known cases and those private cases which in one way or other were in receipt of aid or care. When you examined the registers, however, there were people listed who had not been seen for years but their names were kept on the books. They might even have gone to England and died there and the liaison which we had organised with the British to follow up cases had not worked and we still had them on our lists. In the same way, people who had only a primary lesion on first diagnosis and who had recovered, might still be there on the register. So, we decided to define a 'case' as any person on a tuberculosis register who had had a positive sputum[1] within the previous two years, or whose last available x-rays, taken within the previous two years indicated active disease and that he or she was still in need of treatment. Using these criteria, we reduced the numbers on the registers from 30,000 to 11,642 pulmonary cases and 2,788 non-pulmonary cases, mainly bone and joint. We found

1.   Coughing up live bacilli.

cases which were on more than one register, people who had left the areas, cases who were dead and so on. So in this way, we carried out a national clean-up of the registers and were able to classify the cases on a standardised basis.

Next we began one of the most important parts of the Survey. With the cooperation of the Chief Medical Officers of the cities and counties, each person on the register of every county was examined very thoroughly. They had an x-ray, sputum test or tests and so on so as to bring their clinical examination status up to date. Their social background was carefully examined by the Survey's Almoners, Maureen Reynolds and Theresa MacCann. Dr Bridget Walsh examined the Dublin cases and Dr M.M. Conran did the rest of the country. Nearly 90 per cent of all cases agreed to be examined.

There were 6,000 cases in beds, in sanatoria or hospitals and these I examined myself. All but four agreed to see me and go through the screening procedure. The morbidity part of the Survey took just over a year to complete. Different parts are worth mentioning. First it was far more difficult to do than we thought. TB patients can be as elusive as quicksilver and sometimes it took a long and painstaking chase to catch up with them and secure their cooperation. It was easier to do those in sanatoria, since they were more or less captive. Some were very ill and had to be taken very easily, others were querulous and wanted to know what it was all about and then went over to criticism. One had to have patience and satisfy them as best one could before getting started on the job. It was both monotonous and sad going from bed to bed, but I tried to cheer them up as I went. For most, anything to break the ennui of sanatorium existence was welcome.

When all the material was collected and had been punched onto cards, the analysis began. Certain things stood out. From a total of 10,000 patients coughing up sputum, about one-third were sputum positive to a TB bacillus test and therefore infectious. Of these the vast majority were in sanatoria and unlikely to be able to spread the disease. This showed that the doctors working with TB were on the ball and had so far managed to isolate all the infectious cases they could find. But the disease was certainly active in the community, infection was certainly there and new cases were appearing. Therefore there were infectious cases still at large and spreading it and they remained to be found.

The analysis of the clinical data showed that the majority of cases developed the disease as a simple fever illness with minor symptoms, the sort of thing which could be easily missed. Yet when first x-rayed, although the patient's general condition seemed good, the disease was well established. The length of time between the patient's first feeling ill and the diagnosis of the disease was usually minimal and delay in the diagnosis was infrequent. The Irish doctors knew what they were doing and missed little.

But a very large number of patients exhibited, on first diagnosis, extensive lung damage. In Dublin 50 per cent of all males on being first seen were in categories which exhibited very severe lesions. Of all cases 30/40 per cent showed cavities on first x-ray, or diseased holes in their lungs irrespective of treatment. The proportion was higher amongst males. A quarter of all cases had had some form of surgical treatment in 1951.

The information derived from this part of the Survey showed the extreme difficulty of effecting cures when so many cases already had serious lung damage. You can cut out but you cannot cure a destroyed lung. The number of cases with advanced disease and wide-spread cavitation or big septic holes in their lungs was very large. With earlier diagnosis, a much more favourable result could have been achieved.

We also examined the 2,788 cases of non-pulmonary or bone and joint cases and were satisfied that we got all of them, at least the serious ones, though we may have missed some cervical glands or other minor conditions. The cases showing the maximum incidence and severity were TB spines or Pott's disease and TB hips. The most significant factor in the spread of such forms of the disease was the number of previous cases of tuberculosis in the patients' homes.

Of 8,716 chest cases who were reviewed, only 550 were judged to be capable in the future of undertaking full employment in their previous occupation. From the total of 11,642 persons with lung, bone or joint or both disease, 2,500 might be capable of partial employment. The most difficult part of the problem is the training of unskilled labour, previously engaged in heavy manual work and the provision of suitable employment for them.

Then we went on to study how the disease spreads once it has secured a lodgement in the body. We did this in two ways. One was to look at material that had been removed by chest surgery. It had not been possible to study this properly, till Dr Gough in Llanlough Hospital near Cardiff devised an instrument which enabled us to prepare such specimens for examination. I went to see him and he showed me his technique and we appointed Dr Dermot Holland, then a young and innocent pathologist, who later became Professor of Pathology in the Royal College of Surgeons and ended as the distinguished President of the Royal College of Physicians. Dermot found a high percentage, particularly in young females, of progressing primary lesions. He was able to describe the spread of the disease in the lungs in a way that had not been seen before and to show the body's resistance by calcification and fibrosis. Then he could show the mechanical complications which occur as a result of the tuberculous process following the healing of lesions. For example, a healed lesion might cause narrowing of a bronchus and a collapse of part of the lung. He prepared thinly sliced specimens on large photographic plates and treated them with preservatives, and we showed these to the staffs of the sanatoria. These demonstrated very clearly the relationship between what the patients were experiencing as symptoms, what physical examination showed when one examined the chest and finally what was the x-ray picture of the lesions. These exercises made the work much more accurate all through the sanatorium service. We could see the significance of the cellular response and the prognosis and a lot of other important pieces of information became available in relating the signs and symptoms of the early cases together and to enable us to realise what they meant.

Then we had a look at the tubercle bacillus itself. From the hospitals and sanatoria patients we isolated 903 strains of tubercle bacilli. Of 860 strains from people with lung disease, 1 per cent were of the bovine strain, possibly coming from cattle. Of the bone and joint disease, the majority were human bacilli and only about 10 per cent were of the bovine type. We tried to relate the virulence of the bacilli we grew to the kind of lesions produced but we had little success with this.

However, one could say that we produced the first clear picture of the role of bovine tuberculosis in causing the disease in humans in this country.

The next stage in our activities was to carry out community surveys in two towns and four country districts. We knew that there were active foci of infection which were spreading the disease but we had to learn how to find them. So we went in with our 40 mm mirror-camera mobile x-ray unit and during a short time in each of these places, we x-rayed 18,245 persons. Of these 28 were found to have a positive TB sputum, and 43 persons were sent to sanatoria. Two findings from this exercise were significant. One was that a very small number of infectious persons could keep the disease going, and it was therefore imperative to find these people. The other was that without active follow-up, mass x-ray would not be really successful, because many people recalled because of an abnormality would simply not turn up.

In Dundalk and Dungarvan, the two towns we 'did', we looked at the milk supplies. In those pre-pasteurised days, we found in Dundalk 2,000 cows in 160 herds supplying the town, of which seven herds were found to be producing milk with live tubercle bacilli. In Dungarvan, one herd from 20 herds (460 cows) was producing tuberculous milk.

Next we had a look at the factors favouring the spread of the disease. We took two aspects, firstly factors favouring the spread of infection and secondly, factors lowering the resistance of the individual to the disease.

A lot of material was collected, but a simple account of the results showed that influences operating in the home or family seemed to have been the major factor in the spread of the disease. Thirty per cent of all patients, themselves, blamed infection in their homes. The 3,160 persons who blamed infection in their homes had 4,942 close relatives who had suffered from the disease during the previous ten years. The spread among siblings was notable. We found that the known cases had 38,151 home or close family contacts and it was obvious that this was the most important and the immediate group at risk. We found that there were concentrations of the disease in various employments. In a study of eleven new housing areas in five towns we found that in the previous ten years

there had been a very large number of deaths and of new
cases diagnosed, that opportunities for the spread of infection
were great, that a large population of young people were at
risk and that serious housing over-crowding was occurring.
The urgency of the problem and the necessity for its control
was demonstrated. We also studied stress as a factor affecting
the spread of the disease. Things like unemployment, living in
lodgings, nutrition, housing and other social factors were also
examined, as were racial susceptibility, and the contributory
effects of emigration and migration and alcoholism.

The examination of the cases, the studies on the factors
favouring the spread of the disease and all the rest of it, were
carried out with the cooperation of the County and City
Medical Officers of Health and the specialist TB officers
in Dublin. This had a tremendous effect on the success of the
Survey. Once we had carried out the studies on the deaths
and the known cases in order to define the problem and to
indicate or demonstrate how the tubercle bacillus had secured
a foothold in people's bodies in the community, we went on
to study what might be out there that we did not know.

As I mentioned earlier we surveyed Dundalk and Dungarvan
and the country districts, but we did these surveys as a combined operation in each place. This operation started with a
census of the community in order to establish a base-line which
we could use in relation to the mass x-ray examination. We
tuberculin tested all the children and immunised all negative
reactors with BCG. We carried out an intensive follow-up of
all those recalled because of an abnormal x-ray. Six weeks
later we paid a return visit to evaluate the results.

I must admit to prejudice in the selection of places to study.
I chose Dundalk because I came from the next county, Armagh.
It is a tough border town, where they are hard-headed sensible
people. They do not respect anyone or anything unless it
adds up and makes sense. On the other hand they are warm-
hearted folk and if you can enthuse them into doing something
which they think is worthwhile, they'll do it and do it well.
They were exactly the kind of rough, tough, clever, talented
warm-hearted Irish people I love to work with and with whom
I get on well. I felt that if I could talk them into agreeing
to let me turn their town upside down with my circus, I would
have it made.

People think alike in these things and when later the British followed, doing the same sort of thing on a huge scale, deploying 100 mass x-ray units at one time, they chose Liverpool and Glasgow, two lively genuine towns. I think that they were inspired possibly with the same idea as mine, if the thing would work in Dundalk, it would work anywhere. So far as I know Dundalk was one of the first towns in Europe to get this 'blitz' treatment.

Then I picked Dungarvan as a suitable medium-sized town. Some years before in a residential school, a famous little place where children learnt Irish in a unique way, a diphtheria immunisation programme had been carried out and through a mishap the children were injected with live tubercle bacilli. The matter received world attention as some died. If the prejudice lingering from this incident could not stop us, we could be assured of the success of any mass x-ray campaign anywhere.

Then we went to four country areas. The first was Bansha in Tipperary, where the parish priest was my friend Father Hayes, the Founder of Muintir na Tir (The People of the Land). He had a wonderful parish organisation and we used it. In one hour Father Hayes could have a message in every house in his huge parish. He simply went into his two or three schools, wrote the message on the blackboard in each classroom, each child copied it into his or her exercise book and on the way home from school called into each house as instructed, wrote the message down and left it on the kitchen table; result, instant communication. The whole place was run like this and it was a joy to survey. Then up to Moynalty in County Meath, a mixed village and rural area, then to Tara in the same county, a symbolic place, the ancient seat of the High Kings of Ireland, where in any case the parish priest, Father Cooney, was an old friend of my father's and gave us his backing. Then we went to Ardbraccan, a place where the traditional industry was stonecutting and where the carving of the limestone might have an effect on the lungs of the workers.

In each case we were feeling our way; working out techniques as to how to apply new methods, how to do a 'combined' operation of 1) tuberculin testing, 2) BCG vaccination, 3) mass radiography, 4) sputum testing, 5) epidemiological study, 6) mapping of cases on ordnance survey maps, and 7) follow-up.

We learnt to move into a place, do a census and the public relations in advance of the arrival of the team, then do the job, move on to the next place, which had already been prepared, while the follow-up lot did a kind of mopping up afterwards. We found that with a bit of practice we could be in and out of a place quickly. A raised level of tuberculin positivity in a class in a school meant that we x-rayed the teacher to see whether he or she was infected. On the other hand we might find a child with a flaring primary and infecting his mates which we would follow up to the home to find the initial infecting focus. In a place like Dundalk, to find the infectious cases amongst those who turned up for a check after their x-ray showed an abnormality, was easy, but it was very difficult amongst those who did not turn up, and they were usually the ones we really wanted to get our hands on. The Survey was one great national pilot operation for national TB eradication. All the time we were preparing for a national TB clean-up on the lines we were researching.

In the areas we examined the total population was 31,675 persons, of these 24,464 were examined by mass x-ray and tuberculin testing, which amounted to two-thirds of the total population and 85 per cent of those under 45 years of age. 5,924 persons received BCG vaccination.

We used local community organisations and voluntary labour extensively. In Dundalk for instance we established our headquarters in the hall of the Gaelic League. We harnessed the local Irish Red Cross Unit and their people worked day and night to make the thing a success. We found leaders like Paddy Power, the school teacher and local Red Cross Chief, politicians, socialite leading ladies like Miss Agnes Carroll, clergy, trade-unionists and all kinds of people who were concerned to end this TB scourge. And of course the local doctors, who backed me up. On the other hand one decent man, a very good doctor, fought us tooth and nail, as people invading the privacy of the ordinary man's personality and home. Anyway it worked and as regards TB Dundalk was never the same again. The real thing was that it was the Dundalk people who did all the work.

If you add the whole thing up, we found two or three

things which were enough to end TB in Ireland. One was that when infection occurred, it was pretty deadly. When we cleaned up the registers there were up to 12,000 known cases. One in three of these, almost 4,000 people, died each year from the disease. Most cases were well-advanced on first diagnosis, lung destruction had already occurred and cure in the accepted sense was impossible. There was overwhelming evidence of the manner of spread to close contacts of known cases, who were the people at risk. Relative to the total population their number was small however and if they could be protected, the spread of the disease could be halted to a large extent. The priorities therefore were to find cases early, before the lung damage had occurred, and while the cases were infectious, and to protect the contacts. There were other things. When cases were found on x-ray screening, it was clear that this was only the beginning. Every suspect presented an individual problem. Forty per cent did not turn up for a follow-up check. This phenomenon of patients failing to turn up when summoned for a recall x-ray or defaulting when undergoing treatment, was by no means peculiar to Ireland, as it was later found in other countries. The variety of the failures in response (which we analysed in detail as part of the study) showed the need for effective supervision of cases and suspected cases. This was of importance in the successful use of the anti-TB drugs, which came along a couple of years later. They would not have had anything like the effect expected without the early finding of cases and the effective supervision of patients undergoing treatment.

The Survey confirmed that the disease could be conquered because the numbers were small enough to handle. To do this we had to be able to concentrate the entire forces of the service on to each individual case and his or her contacts in a 'combined operation'. As a result of the research work, we now really knew what we were doing.

There were several minor spin-offs to the Survey. One was that we drew up a national recording chart for all cases, so designed that it was capable of acting as a source of statistical analysis. Another was that we laid the foundations for a National Report Centre, which we established later and which enabled us to monitor the progress of our campaign against

the disease. Another interesting study was a survey of Pneu-
monconiosis or dust disease amongst the miners in Castlecomer,
Co Kilkenny and Arigna, Co Leitrim. In Castlecomer, where
they mined anthracite, we found quite a number of cases of
the disease, particularly amongst the older miners. These
cases were the first described in Ireland. As it was not known
here before and as some of the men were suffering badly, it
raised the question of their compensation. During the course
of the work John Chambers, our bacteriologist, came on atypical tubercle bacilli — the first found. He cultured and recultured
them over and over again but they still retained their abnormal
characteristics. There was an international Symposium on the
Chemotherapy of Tuberculosis in Dublin in 1951 and many
of the delegates came to see our atypical strains and agreed
that we were on to something new. This original discovery has
since been elaborated very considerably by subsequent work.
The last part of the Survey was the report which we submitted
to the Medical Research Council, published by them and distributed in the first weeks of 1954.

In my life, I have had some good periods and some not so
good, but the years I spent with the National TB Survey were
amongst the best.

We were fortunate in having two brilliant radiologists, Niall
Walsh first, who developed the mass-radiography techniques
with Ann Roddy and the other radiographers. When he left to
go to Newfoundland, Joan MacCarthy joined us. She developed
the studies on the radio-pathology involved in the development
of lesions as well as carrying out the MMR work in the Dundalk Survey. We had first-class medical officers, Dr Bridget
Walsh and Dr M.M. Conran who were responsible for the field
work and the surveys in the urban and rural areas. John
Chambers, our bacteriologist, set up a laboratory from scratch,
trained technicians and provided a first class service. The two
secretaries, radiographers, almoners, punch card machinists,
technicians and all the others were a memorable lot and their
names are on the masthead of the Report. The total cost of
the Survey was £50,000.

However, I had some fantastic luck. If I had not attended
the 6th International Congress of Radiology in London in
August 1950, (just after commencing the Survey), the first

such Congress for nearly 15 years, I would not have seen the
first ever mirror-camera mass x-ray unit shown by Schonander
of Sweden. Then with the advice and encouragement of some
Irish radiologists who were present (I remember Drs MacHugh,
Boland, Geraghty and Reynolds), I bought the set off the
manufacturers' stand, brought it home and so had the first
mirror camera unit in these islands.

We started a development programme under Niall Walsh
and Ann Roddy, with training and handling exercises and
when we had learnt enough, I had the set mounted on a Bedford truck, with a body which we designed and had built in
Dublin. We fined it down so that the unit could go anywhere
and be operated with one radiographer and a driver/technician
and could be plugged into any 15 amp light socket, or might
be stopped and used at any cross-roads or in any small school
house. This was essential and ideal for our scattered rural
population. The larger units, I had seen abroad, cost 10/- per
film or per person examined. We got it down to 2/-, more in
keeping with our means. When we finished our R & D work,
we wrote it up and published it in *Tubercle*, the Journal of
the British Tuberculosis Association. It aroused a lot of
interest as it was the first account of the first mirror-camera
unit in Great Britain or Ireland. The successful development
of mass radiography in this country was based on this work.

The second of a whole series of lucky breaks was getting
Montrose. It was a beautiful old mansion, quite empty and
there for us to use. I have many memories of the place. On
the first day we were all there, Father Feichim O'Doherty of
UCD came and said Mass in the hall of Montrose and we asked
for the Lord's Blessing on the work.

To carry out an enterprise like this, it is not enough to do
the thing as a routine job. You have to believe in it, to be concerned, to feel that what you are doing can save lives and
suffering and you have to become dedicated. It is as simple
as that. It may sound corny but we did it, and enjoyed it and
it worked. Lots of other people have done similar things all
over the world and they did not have Mass and still did an
excellent job, but this is the way we felt and it made us happy.
I tell this because to-day, Montrose is the headquarters and
the studios of RTE, the Irish National Television authority. I

sometimes think that the television personalities of to-day should appreciate that a lot of people did quite a job on the same site before they were ever heard of.

As the project came near to its end, people began to look for jobs, and eventually everyone was placed. The prestige of the work helped. Just as I had walked in a single person to start it, so I left as the last survivor and I felt sad that it was all over. On an impulse, I went to the animal houses. There we had a large number of guinea pigs and rabbits, used to detect or type the different strains of the tubercle bacillus.

I found that the chap in charge of the animal house had finished off the miserable creatures in the cages, which was the only thing to be done to those whose lives had been sacrificed that man might live, but lacking instructions on what to do with the bodies and having been paid off and gone to another job, he had left everything. So I spent two days or more burning the hundreds of poor corpses. As they were all pretty rotten with tubercle, they could not be dumped, so I burnt the lot. Every time I go past Montrose, I can still smell the incineration.

One interesting aspect of the National Tuberculosis Survey was the visits from people from all over the world. They included Ministers of Health from African countries, Heads of tuberculosis services in Europe and others. The highlight of these visits was unusual. One day, I think in 1951, my wife rang to say that a Dr Palmer had been on the phone and left a number to ring and that it was urgent. She said that he was an American, that he had been on to the Department and they told him that I did not work there any more, that they did not know where I could be found but that Dr Browne, the Minister would see him. She said that he was all fussed up about something and that I had better contact him.

It turned out that he was Dr Palmer, the Assistant Surgeon-General of the US. He asked me to meet him as soon as possible in the Hibernian Hotel. It was all very mysterious and when I got there he produced Mr Oscar Ewing, the Health, Education and Welfare Administrator, the Government Minister for these matters, in the Democratic Government of President Harry Truman. The President sent Ewing and a plane-load of senior officials from the Surgeon-General's Department to examine the British National Health Service. The visit was arranged by the Rockefeller Foundation, who asked Mr Ewing to take a day in Dublin to see me. We spent most of the day together sitting in the sun on a bench in St Stephen's Green, while they put me through the mill with questions on child health, TB and the organisation of health services. I remember that they stood me a marvellous lunch in the old Russell Hotel. It was all very flattering.

The mass x-ray units of the MMR Company carried out over 2 million x-ray examinations between 1951 and 1960 and for the three years before 1960, averaged 280,000 a year. This was from a population of 3 millions, and when children and the aged are excluded it was a very creditable performance. These results were due to the hard work of Jerry Magnier, formerly a major-general in the Indian Medical Service, then to M.P. O'Brien of Edenderry, who had been in my class at school.

9

Return to the Department

DURING my absence on the Survey, my post was filled by J.D. MacCormack and he carried the medical team through the Mother and Child storm. They were not involved in it to any great extent since as I understand it they rarely saw the Minister or were consulted by him.

John Costello took over after Noel Browne left. I was still finishing the National Tuberculosis Survey so did not see anything of him. From the stories, he was quite different from the others. He worked only with the medical staff, whom he saw all day every day. When he had decided what he wanted to do, he sent for the Secretary of the Department and in the presence of the medical people gave him his orders. As he was Taoiseach as well as Minister for Health and had a positive determined manner, no one dared to say anything, but the administration did not like it.

Later we had Tom O'Higgins, who afterwards became the Chief Justice and after that again a Judge of the International Court in the Hague. He was very proper and a courteous gentleman. I had been a friend of his father who was County Medical Officer for County Meath and a Fine Gael Deputy in the Dail. He was interesting as a member of a distinguished professional family which had espoused the national cause, had suffered for it and now was contributing to the establishment of the new State.

We did not see a lot of him, because he mostly worked through the administrative side. However he too made a positive contribution. Granted that much had been achieved in planning and initiating things before his arrival, it could be said that he did not have a lot to do except to allow the machine to proceed. But when he came in he said that he wanted to establish a voluntary insurance agency and from the start pursued this and brought it to a successful conclusion. It has proved an immense boon, at first to middle-class people who otherwise would find it difficult to meet the cost of hospital and specialist care. Later more and more people have joined as society in Ireland has become 'embourgeoised' and by group schemes and other arrangements a very large section of the population are now covered. It has been a great success. It has had a happy spin-off, in that it has relieved the burden which would of necessity have fallen on hospitals, if everyone came in without having to pay and it has assisted in the cost of providing care for the poorer sections of the community.

Mr O'Higgins was fortunate in that he found a very good man in the Department, Sean O'Mahony, to develop his Scheme. Sean was later appointed General Manager and Chief Executive of the VHI. He left the Department to take it over and eventually made our Voluntary Health Insurance one of the best in the world.

I have given a fairly close account of the period and of my experience under the regime of Dr Browne as Minister. My fate was not unusual. This kind of thing happens to Chief Medical Officers or Advisers all over the world. It is an occupational risk, that is unless you are prepared to keep your head down and do as little as possible, or live at a quiet time with amiable Ministers, or become political yourself. In the Scandinavian countries, this is what they sometimes do, for instance my friend, Johannes Frandsen, the Chief Medical Officer of Denmark, was a member of the Country Party and had a seat in parliament. When I went to New York in 1946, I found that Mayor Dwyer blamed Hugh Stebbins for closing down New York during the tug-boat men's strike, and made him the scapegoat. Hugh Stebbins was Commissioner for Health and later was Dean of the School of Public Health in Johns Hopkins University in Baltimore and a very great man.

The Director of the Health Services in Israel, Simon Btesh, had experiences infinitely worse than anything I had to stand. Simon came to WHO and ended up as Director of the Division of Scientific Research. He told me that for years he carried the psychological scars of that time. He too wrote an auto-biography telling his story.

When I returned to the Department in 1953 I found that

things had changed quite a bit. They were still pursuing the original 1945 programme. We also had the findings of the TB Survey to implement and that was going to take quite a bit of work. Then Dr Ryan had gone ahead with the Mother and Child plan only to run up against the bishops as before. Before my return to the Department he had talked to me about changes which might be acceptable if he was forced to review the programme. I told him that I had only one hang-up about it. So long as the children of the poor were covered that was all I wanted. The vast majority of child deaths were the deaths of the children of the poor. The bulk of defects found in the schools medical examinations were found amongst the children of the poor. I asked him for God's sake to put an end to the nonsense and let us get on with the job of taking care of the children of the people who needed it.

It was all very dramatic and complicated and subject to compromise. Mr de Valera and Dr Ryan met Cardinal Dalton of Armagh (a wise man who was very unhappy about the whole matter) and through him the bishops, and the whole thing was sorted out. In the end we got more or less what we wanted. We were able to provide a good national ante-natal, delivery and post-natal service for most mothers and infants and the care included pre-school children. We got free medical care for school children requiring attention for anything discovered at schools examinations. This was interpreted liberally to cover all children requiring such care and who were attending primary schools. The important thing was that it covered the mothers and children of the poor and of those in large families.

In inaugurating the abridged Mother and Child Scheme I had a pleasant period working with Brendan O'Herlihy, one of the brightest administrators in the service and a good friend. The new scheme gave women a choice of doctor and we arranged that the ante-natal service should be on a fee-for-service basis, set at a decent level, so that the doctors got paid properly for anything they did and were likely to work hard to popularise the service since it was to their benefit as well as to the patient. It was a happy cooperation between the administrative and the medical sides of the Department. James Ryan the Minister gave it his full support. We also set up a 'peer' review of all maternal deaths and acted on the advice given to reduce them. Each death in child-birth was reviewed by a panel of the country's top obstetricians. and was the subject of a report. It was the beginning of a national feed-back on such things. About this time, I did my first cancer reviews, in which I monitored the deaths from cancer over the previous ten years and noticed for the first time that the deaths from lung cancer were beginning to creep up. I also did a study on perinatal mortality, the first on the subject from Ireland, which I published in the *Irish Journal of Medical Science*. So it was a happy time. The medical staff were all busy and the younger men who had come in were turning out very well indeed.

About this time too, I became Chairman of the Institute of Almoners. To take the chair at their meetings usually held after 5 pm and to see these young women, bone-weary after their day's work coping with misery and poverty was an inspira-tion to someone like me. In my job the dreadful danger was of becoming too complacent. We tried to improve their con-ditions of service but their problem of helping people who could not or would not cope with life still remained. I also began to take an interest in the Third World. Half-way through the 1950s it became apparent to people in Europe how appal-ling matters were in Asia and Africa. Through the World Health Organisation and our missionaries, and other sources, we had everyday evidence of the prevalence of tropical diseases, malnutrition, infant deaths, population pressures and so on. Anyone with a social conscience became more and more impressed with the need to do something about it.

This was reinforced by a visit we had from Dr Marcolino Candau, the Director-General of the World Health Organisation and Dr Norman Begg, the Scottish Director of the European Region of WHO. They had heard something of what we were doing and came to see for themselves. Charlie Lysaght and I first took them down the country and showed them some of the hospital building, the new mass x-ray service, and the beginnings of the Mother and Child scheme. In Dublin, we showed them things like the intensive care units for infants and the domiciliary care of the neonatals carried out in places like the Rotunda, and we visited Trinity, the College of Sur-

geons and UCD. At the College of Physicians Dr Candau was
made an Honorary Fellow of the Royal Academy of Medicine.
They were impressed, and Candau asked me would I like to
come to work for WHO. I said that there was a lot still to do
in Ireland. He said that he would like to leave it open.

Smallpox
At the turn of the century Ireland was probably the best vaccinated country in the world; in consequence the last case of
smallpox we had was in 1911 in Athy. Compulsory vaccination
was rigidly enforced. It was one of the responsibilities of the
medical staff of the Department to ensure that the dispensary
medical officers carried out this vaccination and defaulters
amongst the local people were prosecuted in the district courts.
It was customary to read on one page of the local paper of
people being fined for not having lights on their bicycles, and
on another of fines imposed on vaccination defaulters, as they
were known. As so frequently happens, the coming of Independence brought an antagonism to anything made compulsory
by the British and of course this included vaccination. Throughout the country there was widespread evasion. The Irish people
decided that vaccination against a disease that had not been
seen for thirty years was just not necessary.

Now this was one of the few things about which J.D. Mac-
Cormack and my older colleagues and I had quarrels. They
wanted to enforce the compulsory vaccination. This scheme
had been their pride and it was something for which they and
their predecessors had fought hard to achieve. I felt that by
1944, evasion was so bad that it was far better to treat the
whole country as being wide open to smallpox.

There were other complications. We had our own Vaccine
Institute, at Sandymount, owned privately by the Holmes
Denham family of doctors who produced the safest vaccine
anywhere. In a hundred years we had never in this country
had a case of encephalitis, the bane of smallpox vaccination.
It is, however, true to say that the vaccine lymph was very
strong and gave every adult a very large swollen and sore arm
when vaccinated and this prejudiced people against it.

If we were to regard Ireland as being wide open to smallpox,
we had to be on our toes to prevent the introduction of the

disease. Our main problem was ships coming from the East, Latin America, the Middle East, Africa and so on, which did not come here directly but docked in British ports. Passengers coming to Ireland made their way here afterwards. The same thing applied to travel by air. Therefore we monitored the British radio and later the television each night to hear of cases of smallpox coming to Britain. I had an arrangement with the British Ministry of Health, so that they would let us know of any passengers from smallpox infected ships who might be coming to Ireland. It did not work very well, because their system of reporting was not fast enough for us. It was amusing because sometimes we rang and told them. But the Medical Officers of the major ports were first class. These people were on the phone to us immediately a ship came in with a suspected smallpox and would give us the names of people who had an Irish destination. We would then pick them up when they came here.

Depending on the degree of contact we would quarantine them at Clonskeagh Fever Hospital, where we had a national isolation unit under Dr Elcock and a fully vaccinated stand-by staff. In the event of a case they would be locked up with the patient to nurse him or her. The regular vaccination was essential. It was rumoured that one of the largest British ports had neglected to vaccinate their stand-by staff, and when a case was admitted from a ship, some of them became infected and died.

J.D. MacCormack (once I had overcome his resistance) and then Harry O'Flanagan took a great interest in this game. With the coming of television, a smallpox case anywhere in Western Europe caused panic. A case in Moscow ended up in their having to vaccinate seven million people. In an English outbreak, the television showed long lines of people queuing for vaccination and some panic and confusion.

J.D. and Harry became so good at surveillance that a young man who had attended a hospital dance in England and who had danced with a nurse who had been remotely connected with a case, found to his surprise that we had traced him here and he was promptly popped into quarantine in Clonskeagh the next day. Someone coming from the East, if there was the slightest suspicion of contact, would find on his arrival home, that everyone in the house and all those with whom he might come in contact had been vaccinated the day before. We had a panel of elderly doctors who had served in Africa or the East whom we used to look at suspected cases. We had to have these old fellows as no one in practice of the usual doctor's age had ever seen a case of smallpox. Later when Paddy Meenan had his virus laboratory going, he provided a diagnostic service for us. This work of vaccination and the protection of families was the work of the CMOs and they were enthusiastic over it. But they had a problem in that if anyone had told them to 'get lost' or to refuse to go into quarantine there was nothing they could do about it and be within legal limits. The fact that they managed so well was a tribute to their powers of persuasion. Whenever we sought power under the different Health Acts to detain people who were infected or suspected of being infected with an epidemic disease, there was an outcry about our interfering with the rights of the citizen. No doubt the public would have been even more agitated if we had had an outbreak of smallpox, because the disease had penetrated our defences.

WHO secured one of its greatest triumphs in the world fight against disease by eradicating smallpox. Dr Henderson, an American, was given responsibility for the campaign. It was Henderson's great ability, energy and drive which brought the campaign to its final triumph. Every month, Dr Candau the Director-General of WHO had a meeting with the senior staff in Geneva. On one occasion, Dr Henderson was discussing the progress of the world campaign against smallpox and described the millions who were being vaccinated here and the millions there, a colossal task. Being as usual unable to keep quiet on such occasions, I got to my feet and pointed out that we in Ireland had not had a case since 1911, were completely unprotected or largely so and were at the mercy of our neighbours who on occasion could be very slack indeed. I explained that we had adopted a policy of 'containment' and that short of a mass vaccination of the whole country, which wasn't on anyway, it was the only alternative that made sense. I therefore suggested that Dr Henderson might consider 'containment' as an alternative or parallel to the mass vaccination of populations. Everyone sat up and took notice and there is no doubt that 'containment' played a part in the eradication of smallpox. Henderson, who is a great man, was probably thinking of it himself. He should be much more honoured than he is and appreciated, since he is still warm to the touch. The work of Dr Arita, his Japanese assistant was also most noteworthy.

The eradication of smallpox put an end to the mild prolonged nightmare which the thought of its introduction into this country occasioned.

The Institute of Professional Civil Servants

As I said, a change had taken place in the Department. In the early days after its foundation in 1947 things had been pretty informal and the medical staff had considerable freedom of action. Now the administrative side had become fully organised on the usual civil service lines. This meant that a professional officer submitting a memorandum on a technical subject through the Chief Medical Adviser would discuss the matter with his senior colleagues and with the CMA, and then the submission would go to the Secretary with the comments and recommendations of the CMA, representing the agreed professional opinion on this technical subject.

The Secretary would then pass on the memorandum for examination to the lay administrator who dealt with the administrative aspects of the subject. The lay administrator would return the memorandum with the comments of the administrative officers in his division or section to the Secretary, who might then direct the administrative officer to prepare a submission to the Minister incorporating the views of the professional and administrative sides. This would be presented by the Secretary or one of the Assistant Secretaries to the Minister. The Minister might or might not discuss the matter with the professional side before giving a decision. The professional side might not see the submission to the Minister, or if they did might not agree with what had been written.

This protocol had many good points. It provided for the orderly processing of business, and placed the Secretary, who had statutory responsibility as accounting officer, in the proper relationship with the Minister and enabled him to control the work of the Department. It was the way it was always done and anything else was unacceptable.

From the professional point of view the system meant that there was a dominance of the administrative point of view in dealing with technical problems. In a science-based Department this was ridiculous. It meant that an unwelcome proposal from the professional side could be side-tracked by having it 'examined' all over the place, until it finally came to roost someplace and could be forgotten. With a highly technical matter, the administrative side were often competent neither to examine a proposal nor to make an adequate presentation. Even more dangerously, they might think they could and make a mess of it. As well, the administrative side sat at their desks, studied files and had no direct contact with problems on the ground. On the other hand, those who had to deal with problems in the 'front line' using scientific technology, were simply inspectors or advisers. This is not to question the high level of intelligence, the integrity and the industry of administrators. I question the system. The more effective the administrative machine became the more difficult it was, from our point of view, to achieve progress. One might spend a long time solving a public health problem, but then have to take three or four times as long organising the handling of the matter in the Department. The waste of time and energy and the frustration could be prodigious. Still they were the people who had the last word on, say, the urgency of a technical problem. More and more people needed to see every paper, and the time wasted in discussion was wearying. Many of the bright young administrative people were just as fed up with the machine as we were. In fact many of them such as Padraic White now of the IDA, James Ievers of the Incorporated Law Society and John O'Mahony of the Voluntary Health Institution went out and achieved success and distinction in the big cold world outside the Custom House.

One could resort to the short cuts, which annoyed everybody, or create situations so that the administrators would find themselves forced to accept policy lines which ordinarily they might not wish to follow. In the long run this could cause rancour, ill-feelings and a perpetual suspicion of everything that came from the professional side.

In the Department of Health in fact there was generally

the decency, good feeling and mutual respect that ensured that people worked amicably together. But of course the system put a strain even on this good feeling.

The system had a bad effect on the professional staff in all Departments. People reacted differently. Some simply put their views on paper and left it at that. If anything went wrong they were covered and the Minister could not blame his advisers. Others, after a time in the civil service, did as little as possible, saying, 'if that's the way they want it, right!'. Others responded violently to such situations, and wore themselves out in anger and frustration. The system tended to destroy the natural creativity of good professional people, or at least to impair their performance.

The system permeates the local as well as the central government. All over the world, engineers make magnificent managers, yet I have only known two engineers who became county managers, which is nonsense. Equally nonsensical is the fact that all the chief executives of the Regional Health Boards, save one, are administrators — the odd man out is an engineer. With 3,000 or more doctors in the country it would seem possible to find a good public health man who would make a capable Chief Executive. Most other countries find them and use them. So you find that the doctors or engineers who have the knowledge and the professional and technical responsibility for a project, have no authority, while the administrators who are not really responsible on such technical matters, have the authority. The joker in the pack can be the Minister, who is often out of his depth with both lots, but who has the power, which is different from authority. In any event he is at the mercy of the Cabinet, the Dail, the Party, the bosses, lobbyists and possibly local political groups.

In 1953 there were 2,000 higher civil servants and 1,300 senior professional staff. These latter included an extraordinary array of professionals. Architects, engineers, lawyers, doctors, and those associated with them such as draughtsmen, surveyors, valuers, legal clerks, nurses, pharmacists, dieticians, and so on. Within the broad term 'scientists' there were geologists, geophysicists, meteorologists, chemists, veterinarians, pathologists, biologists, bacteriologists and chemical analysts. There were accountants, teachers of all kinds, professors, librarians and archaeologists, musicians, painters, actors, publishers and writers. There was a large group of agriculturists, horticulturists, silviculturists and a host of technical inspectors, of schools, factories, uniforms, navigators and their vessels, aircraft, furniture and the large number of technical persons in the Land Commission. If one added the people in the large number of the state-sponsored bodies, the total would come to several times as many more.

Not only were all these people trained in their professions, but all or almost all had higher qualifications and special experience. They were recruited to the service after they had gained experience and at a much older age than the administrators, which of course meant that their pensions were smaller, nor at that time did they receive the family allowances paid to the administrative side. Many were leaders in their respective fields and their work was recognised internationally. Taking them all together they had played a tremendous part in the making of the new Ireland. There is no field, project, development in this country which has not been influenced, inspired, originated or assisted by the brains, creativity and hard-work of this group. But because they were so much the back-room boys and girls, so diverse, they had no 'clout' in the civil service.

However, for their protection they had formed the Institute of Professional Civil Servants and I became President of this body in 1953. I had the idea of trying to organise a scientific civil service board which would span the Departments and which would lead eventually to the establishment of a proper scientific civil service, a thing which happened later in Britain. In an increasingly technical world, certainly as applied to government, our set-up was an anachronism.

As President of the Institute I tried to do something about the situation. I wrote some articles, one was published in *Administration* and unexpectedly for me, was well received. People in the civil service acknowledged that we had a case. I felt that the chief technical or professional officers in a Department should hold the same executive status as an assistant secretary. We were able to set up a study group with the Association of Higher Civil Servants, who had at that time agreed that there was a problem. On the working party were Roy Geary, the statistician, who had two doctorates in science,

A.E. Went, a distinguished scientist in the fields of ichthyology and mariculture from the Department of Agriculture and Fisheries, an agricultural scientist called O'Brien from the Land Commission and myself. We worked very hard for quite a while and made progress. However we got nowhere because the Department of Finance would have nothing to do with it.

Before I finish this bit, let me quote Dr T.K. Whitaker, former chief of the Irish Civil Service and obviously a reformed character, in a speech in the Senate in 1980. The speech was on a bill establishing the Limerick National College of Higher Education. Dr Whitaker advocated essential public safeguards in third level education. He condemned the Bill for treating NIHE Limerick as if it were a state corporation. He felt that it should be a pioneering Institute needing special freedom and flexibility if it were to succeed in the urgent national objectives of promoting technological changes, studies and skills in a country still too biased in favour of the purely academic. Like all converts, Dr Whitaker put the case well. The country is full of little semi-scientific, semi-political, semi-advisory, semi-administrative bodies, all dancing about on the touchline as they are meant to be. The new Health Research Council seems to be just such a one since it would seem that a large minority has no practical experience of health research. Until, at the core, at the centre of power, there is a proper scientific presence, in a properly structured framework and with responsibility to support the government of this country, the sad, sorry situation will continue.

To get back to the Department of Health. Life at this time was full, interesting and was enjoyable. We, my medical colleagues and I, began to build up different parts of the health service. Sometimes we did this by backing an existing and established unit. For example Adams MacConnel had a good neuro-surgical unit in the Richmond Hospital. He was a pioneer. So we put money into it, made it the national neurosurgical centre and ensured that J.P. Lanigan, the young assistant, a fine young man, should get a decent deal. George Fegan was helped to create a varicose vein clinic, an important centre for Dublin. There was no difficulty in selling this to the administrative people as it had an economic value, in that people could have treatment while they remained at work.

We developed the concept of orthodontia and facio-maxillary surgery which took a lot of doing in the Department as it is a costly item. We managed to get a good Dental Officer, Seaumas MacNeill, and he pushed on the schools dental service and laid the foundation for the fluoridation of water supplies, which was afterwards such a national success.

Mental health had always been a separate shop due to the statutory situation of the Chief Inspector of Mental Hospitals. However Joe Kearney, the holder of the post, was more than willing to meet us and we set up psychiatry clinics in the county and regional hospitals and these worked well.

We needed a Virology Unit, so one time when I was in London I called into the London School of Hygiene to have a chat with Professor Rhodes about it. After we had talked for a while, he said that he had a young man of great promise from Ireland actually studying virology in his laboratory downstairs. So we had him up and it was Paddy Meenan. After some chat, it was put to him, would he like to start a virology unit in Dublin, though there was little or no money in it at that stage for anyone. He agreed and when I got back I paid a visit to the Mother General of the Irish Sisters of Charity in St Vincent's Hospital, who agreed to give him a little room to start him and a few pounds for apparatus. Later he came out to share Montrose with us when the TB survey was in progress, as he needed more space. He was invaluable to us for early diagnosis of virus disease and WHO made him an Influenza Report person. Finally he ended up Professor and Dean of the Medical Faculty and interim President of UCD.

We helped set up and encouraged a plastic surgery unit in St Steevens Hospital under Mr Prendiville, an artist in surgery and one of the great medical Prendivilles from Kerry.

The heart surgery development was interesting. Barry O'Donnell started doing it in Our Lady's Hospital for Sick Children in Crumlin, Dublin. It began with surgery for children with congenital heart defects, and progressed to dealing with people who had 'holes' in the heart or narrowing or stenosis of the mitral valve. As the techniques improved more and more people wanted to get in on the act. This was to a large extent surgical adventureism, as there was no money in it and the number of cases was small. We eventually arrived at a stage where there were 'not enough hearts to go around' all the different units trying to set up. To become good at any technique you must have a sufficient throughput of cases; too small a number of cases meant a lower standard of work. Our idea therefore was to discourage the rush of too many surgeons into this field. This seemed right at the time, but a result was that when heart surgery techniques suddenly blossomed out into surgery for by-pass operations we had not enough centres.

We pulled together all the various rehabilitation organisations into a Council to get them to work in harmony but still preserving their autonomy, and setting up a National Centre at Dun Laoghaire under a really good man, Dr Gregg. To go into a ward and find a half-a-dozen crippled jockeys with broken backs, woke you up to the fact that there were more things needed in medicine than pills or the knife.

We started a special place in Cappagh, formerly a hospital for children with TB bone disease, and this was to become a long-term stay institution for children with chest diseases such as asthma. These were to come from amongst the 7,000 such cases we picked up annually from the schools medical examinations. As well as being treated they would be able to continue their education because school facilities were provided.

All these new departures were operated on a shoe-string. Finding a corner in an existing institution, getting the right man or woman to start the unit and giving them their head, worked and worked well. We may have had the ideas and given projects a push and encouragement, but it was the ability and hard-work of those concerned which made them so successful. We were seeking constantly to establish centres of excellence.

Generally during this time we organised the specialist services so that even the most remote part of the country had a full range of specialist clinics, such as ophthalmic, oto-laryngologic, orthopaedic, oncological, psychiatric, paediatric, in addition to good specialist medical, surgical, obstetrical, gynaecological, radiological, anaesthetic services. We also developed a really good laboratory service. In addition, we had physiotherapy at the county level, the special nursing required for neonatal, paediatric and orthopaedic care, radiography and other ancillary services.

We took a hand in developing anaesthesia, working with Tom Gilmartin, afterwards the first Professor and first Dean of the Faculty of Anaesthesiology in the Royal College of Surgeons, and had a fruitful collaboration in training and appointments, until we had a well-trained cadre of specialist anaesthetists.

An interesting feature of development was in the field of pharmaceutical and radiological supplies. As I said, the dispensary service had grown a bit archaic in some ways, and one of these was in the matter of drugs and equipment. In 1944 a colouring material favoured by some of the older men, entitled 'Dragon's Blood', was still on the official list. Once the War was over and things began to move again, I found that there was a cartel of drug companies which operated in such a way as to make the cost of medical supplies to this country more than say 25 per cent higher, than elsewhere.

We had a very able pharmacist in the Department, Shane O'Neill, and the Department of Local Government operated a system called the Combined Purchasing Scheme. For all local authority purchases from a steam-roller for the roads to aspirins for dispensaries, contracts were made with suppliers and prices determined on a basis of tenders. Now if a county council could beat the contract price, then it could buy wherever it liked. But otherwise it purchased all supplies from the official contractors. This scheme was operated for the Department of Local Government by a Mr MacLoughlin, who was highly competent, was first-class at his job and a decent man.

First Shane O'Neill and I revamped the dispensary drug list. I was fresh from general practice and knew what I was doing about medicines, and I sought advice from many people. Then, laying down British Pharmacopeia Standards, we invited bids from suppliers all over the world. This caused an outcry from the doctors and particularly the pharmaceutical companies' drug representatives, who found supplies coming from unexpected sources and they did not like it. Then we got a new source of x-ray film and this angered the radiographers. We had a very good Radiological Adviser Dr Reynolds and he checked on each complaint and usually found them to be groundless. Eventually we broke the cartels and ended up with the cheapest drugs of any health service in Europe, and they were all up to BP standards.

But we went further and gave preference, other things being equal, to materials of Irish manufacture and after a bit, we had places like Antigen in Roscrea, employing hundreds of people, exporting to countries all over the world and laying a firm basis for the present thriving Irish pharmaceutical industry. Dr Gus Jennings took it over from me and with Shane O'Neill and Mr MacLoughlin pushed it a lot further. Companies such as Fannin's started to manufacture hospital equipment. People became interested and the ability of the Irish business men and women did the rest. In a few years, Antigen were supplying WHO, UNICEF, and the Crown Agents and governments everywhere, because their products were good, their prices right and they kept their word on deliveries. The first time I went to India in 1956, I found that they were paying nearly 10/- a gramme or some such price for strepto-mycin while we bought it for 2/-.

On the subject of drugs abuse, I was unhappy that the five or six doctors or nurses who took to morphia or cocaine in any year might end up in the police-court and be destroyed for life without ever being given a chance. So by arrangement with the Commissioner of the Gardaí, the matter was left to us. Every pharmacist in the country maintained a Drug Register and every prescription for addictive drugs was entered. These were carefully maintained and regularly supervised by Shane O'Neill, so if any doctor was writing an unusually large number of such prescriptions we were on to him at once. In the hospitals, there were locked dangerous-drug cupboards, and drugs were not released except on the say-so of some senior with the authority. The maintenance of these controls was the subject of our medical inspectors' regular checking. Further, Shane O'Neill had sole control of the opiate supplies to pharmacists. At that time there were no other outlets. So the thing was pretty well sewn up.

I made an arrangement with Dr Norman Moore of St Patrick's Mental Hospital in Dublin, that he would look after anyone we sent to him. Moore, a humane man and a very good doctor, worked wonders with these people. We also looked after them in other ways. If they were in debt, as they usually were, we arranged with the county manager and their bank manager to handle their creditors and arrange for payments, secured the cooperation of their wives and families and generally tried to take care of them and more particularly made sure that they did no harm to patients.

Dr Hourihan had a deep interest in deaf children and pursued this work in Cabra School and elsewhere. So much so that after the Netherlands, our training for these children was the next best in the world. To see a ballet being performed by children who were stone deaf, using some sort of vibration, was wonderful. Dr Hourihan was invited as a consultant on deafness by the US Government.

Dr Michael Daly was very busy indeed with tuberculosis and was constantly on the alert in finding inefficiency. I remember one such instance where he found that failure to fill beds immediately on patients being discharged, was wasteful. Across the whole system as many as 300 beds might be empty, equal to a large institution. He tightened this up to such an extent that we used to make fun of him and say that he had it so tight, that as a patient got out of one side of the bed, someone new stepped in on the other.

Dr Harry O'Flanagan became dedicated to the cause of poliomyelitis. Before the days of immunisation, he developed in Cherry Orchard Fever Hospital a rescue ambulance for cases where respiration was threatened. This was equipped with an 'iron lung' and a specially trained staff including a fast driver, and could speedily pick up a case anywhere in the country and was a real life-saving effort. He was linked closely to the Copenhagen group and the application of techniques worked out there by anaesthetists during their great polio epidemic, and which he applied to Cork during the serious epidemic there in 1956, undoubtedly saved a great many lives.

Gus Jennings worked with Charles Lysaght in the building of the hospitals but his main interest was in equipment. He was responsible for the organisation of a central hospital laundry for Dublin and for a centralised sterilisation system for all surgical equipment. Malachy Powell, amongst his other exploits, monitored the milk and cattle of Kerry for the fallout, about a month after the first nuclear bomb was tested, in 1960 or so, I cannot remember. I was happy that we were in between the US testing ground over the desert in the west and the USSR on the other side of the Urals and felt that we were safe. But to make sure Malachy teamed up with Dr Russell of the British Agricultural Research Council, who was interested in what we might find. It seemed that when an explosion occurred the particles soared away up to the stratosphere, swirled around and then were fairly evenly deposited, so that we got as big a dose of 'fall-out' as anyone else in the Northern hemisphere. Malachy came to know a great deal about nuclear medicine, and of course for years before we had been monitoring and ensuring the safety of radio-isotopes used in clinical procedures in hospitals. We organised wing-tip containers on aeroplanes for the transport of such materials.

I have described some of the interests of my colleagues as examples of the kind of things we did. These were a few that I remember, but in addition they all had broad responsibilities for counties or cities, for inspections, counselling, planning and general public health activities. Looking back on it, after thirty years and more and with the knowledge of what I have seen in many other countries, they were a wonderful team.

Shortly after I came to the Custom House, I did a study on cancer deaths in the country for the ten years 1936 to 1945. It was revealing and gave a clear picture of the problem. Again, ten years later, from 1946 to 1956, I had another look at it. So I monitored cancer deaths over twenty years. It was interesting to see the changes that had taken place in the first ten years. There was a decrease in stomach cancer, which I could not explain. Cancer of the mouth, jaw, and tongue also decreased markedly and was due to better mouth hygiene and more particularly to a good dental service and facio-maxillary surgery. Skin cancers of the head and neck were also well reduced in number. In the past elderly fishermen, drivers of horse-drawn vehicles and people exposed to the wind and the rain for a life-time and who possibly did not wash too often were particularly subject to rodent ulcers and other skin cancers. There was a great reduction in such cancers as a cause of death. This was due mainly to the new effective treatment for such conditions.

However the most important thing to emerge from the monitoring for my first ten years, was the sudden increase in deaths due to cancer of the lung. It was a most extraordinary thing to find. In the ten years they increased three-fold. I could not understand it at the time, but it was a warning of what was to come. Since then, deaths from cancer of the lung have become so frequent as to become a public health nightmare.

During these years I also did a study of the National Bill of Mortality. For one thing, the streptococcus suddenly seemed to lose its virulence and a whole host of diseases caused by this organism commenced to disappear. Scarletina, a deadly fever disease when I was a boy, had gone. It still existed for a time, but instead of children being seriously ill, they ran around as usual and it only became apparent that they had been infected when mothers noticed that the scarf skin started to peel. This had formerly been a sign of the disease. Rheumatic heart disease each year had caused up to 5,000 deaths in Ireland, mainly among young adults and as a cause of deaths, over a few years it disappeared. Formerly, a feared occupational risk for surgeons and pathologists was that they might prick their finger from a needle or a bone spicule, receive an infection from a virulent streptococcus and this would spread up the arm and within 48 hours they could well be dead from a general septicaemia. This did not happen any more. Erysipelas went too and so did many outbreaks of epidemic sore-throats, many of which led to a rheumatic heart disease afterwards. At one time, we helped organise a monitoring service under Dr Paula O'Connell, for the hundreds of Dublin school-children who developed the condition. We even treated many of them with regular doses of penicillin as a preventive measure to prevent the heart disease. Other conditions, like strepto-coccal infection in childbirth, puerperal fever, which had carried off innumerable women down through the ages, also disappeared.

It was apparent that people were living longer. It was also clear that fewer deaths were occurring between the age of 1 year and 45 or 50 years. With the improved child care and the reduction of TB and the better general practitioner and hospital services, young people were simply not dying the way they used to. The situation was improving all the time and was likely to go on doing so. Of course the standard of living improving helped immeasurably; education, hygiene, even things like refrigerators in people's homes all played a part. But in specific diseases, which were tangible, clear-cut entities,

improved medicine was significant. This was particularly satisfying to us doctors. The study showed that old people were
living longer and remained healthy and that when they died,
the reason was not a single straightforward specific cause, but
more often a pattern of causes associated together, as one organ
after the other wore out and gave up.

In 1954/5 I did a study on perinatal mortality in Ireland. I
analysed the perinatal deaths for the three lying-in hospitals,
where there were exact and defined figures and related them
to the whole country. I showed that the deaths fell into three
groups and that it would be possible to reduce them considerably even with the resources then available. As the services of
the Mother and Child Scheme proceeded and became increasingly effective we expected a very substantial reduction to
take place and this is just exactly what happened. The study
was presented to the Section of Public Health of the Royal
Irish Academy of Medicine in May 1955. There was a distinguished audience to hear it, which included Professor Ira
Hiscock, the President of the American Public Health Association. My great friend Austin Harbinson, the CMO of Dublin
and one of the original pioneers of public health in Ireland,
was Chairman. For me, this was a great occasion. I mention it
for a number of reasons. It was taken seriously, was well-
discussed, was attended by the Masters of the three lying-in
hospitals, by the leading paediatricians and others. It was the
kind of thing I had been seeking for years; if it did nothing
else, it might get the obstetricians and the paediatricians talking to one another. Up to that time, many obstetricians would
not allow the paediatricians across the threshold of the labour
ward. They had to wait till the obstetrician was good and
ready to hand the child over to their care. To-day, you have
neonatal specialist officers. The concept of perinatal mortality
was quite new. It included all infant deaths taking place from
the time of viability of the unborn child, at that time, 28 weeks
(now it is less), through the birth to the end of the first week
of extra-uterine life. The concept was first mentioned at a
Conference at Brussels in 1953 and the European Regional
Office, and the Geneva Headquarters of WHO set up a working party to consider it and they published their report in
1954. This was an entirely new way of looking at what for

the ordinary human being is the most difficult and dangerous period of their entire life. The concept has revolutionised our approach to the reduction of infant mortality.

From 1926 to 1930, the infant mortality rate for Ireland was 70 deaths per 1,000 live births. In the post-war years from 1946 to 1950, once we had ended enteritis, we got it down to 56. In 1954 it was 39. The reduction of 17 between 1950 and 1954 meant the saving of 1,000 babies' lives each year. It is nice to think that the work we started has borne fruit and our successors have done a magnificent job and the reduction has gone on and it has been brought down to 10, one of the lowest in the world.

10

Fresh Fields

A T THE end of 1955, Theo MacWeeney wrote to me from
WHO New Delhi to ask me if I could find someone who
would go to Ceylon and do a national TB survey there. They
wanted something on the lines of our survey in Ireland.

I enquired around, but no one who could do it was interested
in going to Sri Lanka. So, partly because I had begun to have
the feeling that I was becoming a 'stuffed shirt' and partly
because I had a growing sense of compassion about the Third
World, I said that if I could get leave of absence I would do it
myself. It was only when I got to New Delhi that I found out
that this was what Dr Mani, the Regional Director in India,
was after.

Mr MacEntee gave me six months leave of absence, which
on the one hand was very decent but on the other was very
short to do a national survey. I had the uneasy feeling that the
bureaucracy were glad to see me off for a bit. Anyway early
in the spring of 1956, I got my 'shots' and started off.

I went first to Geneva where I was solemnly inducted as a
WHO staff member and briefed with extraordinary kindness
and care. The briefing was not up to much but the kindness
was all important. Everyone going off on a mission like this is
always scared and disturbed. Here was I, putting my reputation,
for what it was worth, on the line by taking on a national survey in a country I had never seen, working with people I had
never known, in a place I had never been, about to use techniques which I did not know would work.

When we got down to work in the Regional Office in New
Delhi, I found that the terms of reference of the proposed survey were not based on up-to-date sampling techniques or on
the use of mass x-rays, which I could accept and I told them
so. That set them back a bit. Eventually they invited me to

write my own, which I did. After a little argument and a little compromise they agreed to them. I found that WHO had had international consultants working in Sri Lanka before on tuberculosis.

After New Delhi I made my way to Sri Lanka. By this time I had become accustomed to the heat. When I got there I found the TB situation disturbing. The Director of the TB service, a fine man and an excellent physician, was mainly interested in the clinical treatment of the disease and was not sure that he really wanted a survey. A WHO consultant was sitting in the main clinic, working out his contract, which it seemed was not going to be renewed. Things did not look too encouraging.

The Director-General of the Health Services, Dr Kahawita, did want a survey, had met me before in Geneva and treated me as one of the brethren of the CMO's trade union. I found that they had a wealth of equipment donated from all over the world or that they had bought themselves. They had a mobile x-ray unit, of the wrong kind, which had never been out of Colombo, but which was quite workable. They had two more on order which had not yet been delivered.

The Colombo doctors were very rich, lived in beautiful houses, and were most hospitable and friendly. A Dr Chellapah, as his life's work in Ceylon, created a Corps of Health Inspectors. This corps was excellent. One could encounter one of these characters when driving along a jungle road, usually beautifully turned out in a starched uniform. He might take you to the Health Office, usually on the verandha of his house, and show you local maps, pin-pointing cases of infectious diseases, his water-supply programme or housing programme and then take you to see the things in action. They were really first-class. Unfortunately they had little or nothing to do with tuberculosis, which was handled by its own largely autonomous organisation.

The Government of Ceylon had a first-class statistical unit under a Cambridge senior wrangler and with better equipment than we had at home. They were not fully occupied and so agreed to help me. I decided to do a random sample survey, based on a system of 50-house blocks, a sampling technique which the Japanese had just perfected. We first did a test-run of 25 blocks of 50 households to test the range of variations, the feasibility and techniques. I then punched through a survey proper of 50 blocks scattered on a mathematically random basis all over the island.

The purpose of the exercise was to determine how much tuberculosis they had, how it was distributed and how it was spreading, all essential knowledge. When we knew this it would be possible to draw up a strategy to deal with their problem.

The trouble here was the same as most other places, that they were trying to cure TB and even though they went through the motions of preventing it, they didn't really know how.

We started training the teams on the existing mass x-ray unit but they told me that they could not take it out of Colombo, that it had never been out as it was too big to pass through the rock arch on the road to Kandy. We took it out and the indefatigable health inspectors let air out of the tyres and it went through with an inch to spare.

There were a variety of small problems to be solved before we could begin. For example, the water in the TB headquarters in Colombo was too hot and dirty to allow us to develop the x-ray films, particularly miniatures, satisfactorily, so I got 3 oil-drums, filled them with sand and gravel from the beach and made a filter. Then I got ice from the cold-store that the British had built in Colombo during the last war and cooled it. It was a 'Heath Robinson' bit of apparatus but it worked.

Our method of survey was a development of the Irish technique. Each mass x-ray unit had three teams attached. One team went ahead and prepared the designated block of 50 houses. This was possibly a village, part of a small town or a few streets or part of a street in a large town or city. The team defined the boundaries, numbered each house, did a census of the residents, gave them numbered tickets and told them what the survey was all about.

Then the unit moved in with the second team and people came to be x-rayed by house-number and these numbers were checked off and those who, for reasons such as sickness, did not turn up were carried to the unit. This group sometimes caused problems but was of particular importance since it usually contained proportionately more cases than the rest of the population.

The spools of x-ray film were taken to headquarters and

read. After the examination the results were communicated to the third team which moved in to 'mop-up'. They took laryngeal swabs from persons showing abnormality on the miniature x-rays. They organised the transport of new-found cases to selected hospitals. Suspected cases were handed over for further investigation by the TB service. Tuberculin negative contacts were given BCG vaccination. In a kind of leap-frog procedure, the first team replaced the third as they advanced. The operation was highly successful but extremely hard work, for the WHO team as well as for the locals.

Our people received great hospitality in the areas they surveyed and the atmosphere was delightful. I experienced the pleasure and the discomfort of sleeping in kajan (palm-leaf) huts, of eating the lovely Ceylon foods, especially the hot curries and the fruits and of enjoying this wonderful land of spices, flowers and incense. I also gained other insights into Sri Lanka's life.

The Singhalese women wear the kandy sari. It is pleated at the side and they have a bare mid-riff and a bodice. They do not carry handbags and their personal possessions were tucked away in their bodices. After reading thousands of x-ray films I became an authority on what Singhalese ladies carried in their bodices. I had a collection of these x-ray films showing all kinds of weird objects and as a public relations exercise, used to project them in the villages at night and it always got a laugh. It exorcised any fears that the people might have had of our invasion of their village.

When we x-rayed a village the Buddhist priest was usually very much in evidence. Afterwards he might consult me on some illness or perhaps we would walk around his temple and I would admire everything, particularly his little stupa or domed structure containing a relic of the Buddha. As a gesture of friendship he would present me with a mango. It was a delightful experience, the simple austere monk in the yellow robe, me an old Irish pirate, enjoying one another's company in the tranquility of the evening, one gentleman to another, humanity and the serenity of the things of the spirit at work.

Even in this lovely island, race and religion generated conflict. We had to be careful that we only used Tamil staff in Tamil villages and Singhalese staff in Singhalese villages. Coming from the North of Ireland I was sensitive to such issues. One time, I was being driven into Colombo from the Galle Face Hotel during a Tamil Satygrha or peaceful sit-down protest. A group of Tamils had marched the several hundred miles from Jaffna and had set themselves down in front of the Parliament House on the green. The mob came out from Colombo and we ran into them. They closed in on us in a frightening way and I thought that they might overturn the car. Suddenly all four doors were opened and they called in, 'Are there any Tamils in this car?' My driver shouted back 'No! we're all Singhalese'. They burst out laughing when they saw my red Irish face and then shephereded us through the crowd. They then went back and threw the poor Tamils into the ornamental lake in front of the Parliament House. Fortunately it was only a shallow ornamental affair and no one was drowned.

I got the job done, including a reorganisation plan for the tuberculosis service, which Dr Kahawata asked me to present at a meeting of the Society of Sri Lanka Medical Officers of Health. Then I said goodbye to the health inspectors, who gave me as a gift a silver tray shaped like the island of Ceylon. I gave a dinner party for my friends and very sadly started on my way home. I went first to New Delhi, where they would not believe that the survey was done, and done well, and then to Geneva where I had a pleasant few days and found myself in the company of some international TB experts. The project which had frightened the wits out of me originally turned out to be not so fearsome. This was not due to me but to the Sri Lanka people who did the work and who worked harder than anyone could have expected.

We had shown incidentally that this survey technique, which we had worked out in Ireland, could be applied to a developing country. We found that they had not nearly as much TB as they thought, that it was in pockets in certain places, and that the main reservoir was amongst the older women who were keeping it going. This was interesting since Sri Lanka is one of the few places in the world where women die younger than men. In the plan, I recommended that if they started an active case-finding effort with follow-up and particularly if they combined it with their excellent public health service, they would certainly surmount the problem.

As a side interest, when surveying the seventy-five sample districts, I had a look at their nutritional situation. Sri Lankan agriculture could then (1956) have been divided into three. A large part was still in natural forest, another large part was in tea, rubber and coconut plantations or cash crops. The remaining third, under rice, was not enough to feed the people and rice had to be imported. At times, if rice could not be landed due to bad weather or strikes in Colombo Harbour, it could happen that there might only be a week's supply of food in the country.

There was a considerable amount of malnutrition to be seen, particularly among the poorer people in Colombo, amongst children of large poor families and in areas where Malaria was present or severe. I reported all this to the Nutrition Section in Geneva and they were interested and took it up with the Government of Sri Lanka and started a nutrition programme for them.

When I got home, I found that J.D. MacCormack was about to retire. I had known it for some time and had asked that his service be extended, but in those days no mercy or compassion was shown to the medicals. To see him go was a wrench as we had become very good friends. He was a great man and should be remembered. His work on diphtheria, begun before the Second World War, was a very fine achievement and must have saved a great many lives. During the time from 1944 to 1956 when he retired, he was indefatigable as a public health man and as our leading epidemiologist.

British Somaliland

In 1957 the WHO at Geneva invited me to do a study on tuberculosis in Liberia. This time I was granted leave of absence for three months only. When I got to Geneva they had changed their minds, and asked me if I would go to British Somaliland instead.

Since Somaliland was a 'hardship' station and accommodation for people like me was primitive, Brian Hughes and his wife Mary Lahart from Holycross in Tipperary made me welcome in their home. Throughout my stay they showed me warm hospitality and unequalled kindness. It was all so long ago but that kindness remains in my memory.

The country was almost entirely desert and was inhabited by four great tribes and some lesser groups. These tribes were a pastoral people and moved in a constant north/south axis up and down the country with their flocks of fat-tailed sheep, goats and camels. The tribes had their own wells and around each were a few mud houses so as to constitute a little town. They were quarrelsome and contested their territories fiercely with their neighbours. These people travelled great distances daily in search of any pasture available in the stony desert and lived hard primitive lives. The Somalis were extremely handsome, tall and spare, were learned in the Koran but were otherwise illiterate, without any visible culture and were tough, fierce and independent.

The capital was Hargeisa, with a miniature British colonial government structure, a legislature, courts and a secretariat. In addition, there was a hospital, a few shops of sorts, the residences of the colonial administrators, a British club and a barracks for a battalion of the Somali Scouts, a unit in some way related to the Kings African Riflers. They had a Governor, Sir Theodore Pyke, who formerly played Rugby for Ireland and was one of the distinguished family of the Rector of Holy Cross in Co. Tipperary.

Berbera, the second town, was a port on the Red Sea, dating back to biblical times. It had a general hospital and a most unusual mental hospital. There were a few more scattered towns, each with a mosque, a small hospital, a few odds and ends of things like a police station and the remainder little mud houses.

A few years before WHO had had a mission in the country consisting of a few Danish and Norwegian nurses to carry out a tuberculin testing survey in the towns. The results had shown one of the highest rates in the world. The government and WHO wanted to know more about it: hence my visit.

The first day, I went to the local TB hospital in Hargeisa and started to examine all the patients. This was by arrangement with the government health people. No one paid much attention to me, and eventually I realised that the staff and patients were 'stoned' out of their minds. About once a week, a convoy of trucks would make it across the desert from Harar in Ethiopia, loaded with bundles of 'kif', a plant of the tea family and a narcotic, something like marihuana. When it came the whole town would go on a 'high'. If the police could get to it first, the smugglers would be hauled before Brian Hughes, the Irish judge in the Hargeisa Court, and fined heavily. I went to the court one day, and the place was heaped up with bundles of hay-like stuff, 'the evidence'.

When I checked on the situation in Hargeisa, I started out across the desert in two land-rovers with Dr Palmer, a very pleasant, knowledgeable and enjoyable travelling companion, who was Deputy Director of the Medical Services, and we went to all the other centres in the Territory. We made our way to Erigavo, a little town right up at the tip of the horn of Africa. It is high up on the great Somali bluff that runs all along the south shore of the Red Sea. We then went down to the border with Italian Somaliland. At each of the more important wells supplying the larger tribes there was a medical post and a medical orderly in charge. I examined the records they kept, but they did not seem to do a big business. The usual entry was an aspirin for a headache or, more important and effective, a thumping big dose of Epsom salts for a constipated tribesman.

The Somali medical assistants in the small hospitals were very good indeed. For example, in the previous year they had diagnosed more than 1,000 cases of TB by the microscopic examination of sputa. The Somali tribesmen walking great distances every day in the hunt for pasture, develop great ulcers on their legs and the medical assistants in the little local hospitals, not medically qualified in a formal or legal sense but highly intelligent, well-trained and skilled had become very expert in skin-grafting these ulcers.

We next had a look at the tribes on the march. Flying into Hargeisa and looking down from the plane, I was struck by the number of 'rings' which were clustered here and there on the ground. I could not recognise what they were. When I went out into the desert, I found that they were rings of great thorn bushes. The moving tribes brought their flocks inside these bush rings at night for protection from such predators as leopards. They also erected their houses inside. These were called 'gurgis' and consisted of large mats made from woven or plaited rushes or some such material. The mats were about 10 feet long by 4 to 5 feet wide. They erected a framework of light springy pieces of wood and laid the mats on this to make a kind of beehive shaped structure. The men seemed to be constantly on the move, ranging ahead looking for a bit of good grazing. Meanwhile, the women loaded the mats and frames on camels, hopped up and along to the next camp site, while the youngsters herded the sheep and goats. Their domestic equipment was a few pots. There seemed to be a lot of spears about.

It was a hard, dry, dusty, dirty, tough life. Most days they seemed to cover from 20 to 25 miles. Occasionally one would come across a great herd of camels being driven down into the Haud desert. The young men with the camels had a few spears, a small bag of millet and a bucket into which they milked the camels. This equipment, with a long strip of cloth to wind around their heads in a dust-storm or to use to try to keep warm at night, was all they had to enable them to spend possibly months with the camels in the desert.

I found a simple explanation for the high incidence of tuberculosis in the towns. A tribesman or woman contracting tuberculosis would be unable to keep up with the families on the march, and would rest up in the towns associated with their particular tribe. There they would be cared for by their kinsmen, at least to some extent. This concentrated the disease in the settlement and caused it to spread amongst the townspeople.

It was therefore important to diagnose it early and to get the cases in for treatment in time, before they could spread the disease further or become too ill. Too many of the available beds in their small sanatoria were occupied by long-term patients. I took a dislike to this lot. They were an arrogant crowd who were in because of their tribal position or because they knew somebody or bribed somebody. It was necessary to find accommodation elsewhere for these people, so as to free beds for early, acute and curable cases. At the same time I was not impressed by the organisation for the supply of drugs by the colonial administration.

After a couple of months hard work, ably assisted by the colonial medical service officers, a report on the situation was

prepared. Our plan consisted in making the tuberculosis service more mobile and not waiting until people broke down
and had to seek refuge in the towns, by which time they were
usually too far gone for anyone to be able to do anything
for them. The question was how? In all these kinds of problems, the answer is usually staring you in the face. Driving
through the desert one would occasionally come across a
character wandering along, wearing a scruffy looking uniform
and leading a camel. These were veterinary 'illaloes', who followed the tribes all over the place and for a small fee injected
the camels against some disease or other. They had been highly
successful, and there seemed to be no reason why the medical
orderlies posted at the wells and peddling doses of salts could
not be sent out after the tribes to look for people with coughs
and sputa and to check the relatives of those who already had
the disease and were in the towns. Anyone they found could
be brought to Hargeisa, Burao or Berbera, where they had
hospitals with x-ray sets and microscopes. If they had the
disease treatment could be started immediately. With a bit of
organisation, they could give babies BCG. In spite of the lives
they lead, the Somalis are intelligent, quick-witted people. In
any case they loved injections, and as this was a national characteristic, BCG protection could be given.

One of the difficulties of a short-term assignment such as
this is that there is no way of knowing that what you recommend will be put into practice once you have gone. But in a
most unusual way, I did find out that something was done.

When visiting the little town of Erigavo, up at the north-
eastern end of the territory, I was taken in charge by a young
Somali health inspector. He brought me around, taking me
into houses to talk to people, showing me the water-supply
he had installed in the mosque for ritual purposes and finally
we ended up at the top of the minaret. When I got back to
Hargeisa, I recommended to Dr Thom, the Scots Director of
the Health Services, that he should send him to England to
get proper training. It was clear that he would be a most valuable native assistant.

Years after, during a session of the Assembly of WHO at
Geneva, I passed a group of Africans chatting away to one
another. One of them broke away, rushed over, threw his arms

around me and then led me over to his friends and introduced me, saying that I was the person responsible for lifting him out of Erigavo and getting him his start in life. He was now the Director of the Health Services for the new Republic of Somalia. He said that he had dug out my report, put the recommendations into operation and that it had worked well.

After this trip I was very glad to come home and to settle down again in my old chair in the Custom House. However I had hardly time to warm it up again, when I was invited to act as one of WHO's representatives speaking for Public Health on a joint World Expert Committee on Nutrition with FAO or the UN Food and Agriculture Organisation in Rome.

Custom House 1957-58

About this time, I was asked to act as Chairman of a European Symposium on Child Health in Berne. It was organised by the European Office of WHO and had people there representing all the European countries. At that time, there was quite a controversy between the two methods of immunisation against poliomyelitis. There was the method of injecting an immunising dose 'the Sabin', and the other was the 'Salk', an oral method. The Czechs had had the sense and courage to go ahead and test the Salk method on a national basis and my Vice-Chairman, a Czech lady in charge of maternity and child health there in their ministry, sitting beside me told me all about it. They had just finished the programme and she had been very much involved and was itching to talk to someone about it. Czecho-Slovakia was the first country to really try the procedure and there had been 100 per cent success. It was so simple, a drop of the agent on a lump of sugar. I followed up her information while I was there, and she sent me on more to Ireland. I became convinced that we might also apply the methods and that the answer to poliomyelitis was now available.

When I got home and sold the idea in the Department, we then contacted the Connaught Laboratories in Toronto, whom we had used for the supply of biological materials for years, always with satisfactory results. We were fortunate in that they had just completed the preparation and testing of this product, so we went ahead and after the Czechs were probably the next of the countries to be immunised against polio. However, we had barely begun the campaign and only a few thousand children had had their doses when a call came from Toronto to say to hold everything. There had been some sort of delayed response from a test on a single monkey and a reaction had occurred which had worried them. There was even a remote possibility that the immunising material could be carcinogenic. Now this is where responsibility of the CMA comes in. No Minister of Health and no administrator can have the knowledge, the judgement or the experience to accept responsibility for an immunisation programme where tens of thousands of children are being dosed with a preventive vaccine like BCG or poliomyelitis or whatever. Yet the person in the Department who really takes the decision and who in the final outcome must accept the responsibility is simply a technical adviser. On occasions he may find it difficult even to see the Minister. After a few days, however, it became apparent that there was nothing wrong with the monkey and the fuss evaporated and I was able to sleep peacefully again.

No matter how you 'pass the buck' or hide behind Committees the decision finally rests with one person. From that one person the responsibility stretches down to the doctor or nurse performing the immunisation. The responsibility does not come down through the administrators or the Chief Executives of the Health Boards. The procedures have to be correct in method and technique.

Then you must be satisfied with your distribution. During my time in Indonesia, BCG vaccine was prepared in a WHO laboratory in the Phillipines and flown to Jakarta. The distribution was in the hands of UNICEF and was their responsibility. Some of the Indonesian doctors got a bit worried about it and complained to me. I investigated its efficiency and found that it was 60 per cent useless due to transport/storage/climatic factors. Once I had established this it was possible to remedy the causes.

Then you must be satisfied with the technique of application. When one considers the daft, careless, crazy things that people can do with drugs, vaccines and sera, it is necessary that the application at the local level is completely fool-proof.

Anyway, we got off our mark quickly with our polio campagn. It worked really well and the results were good. It was the responsibility of Dr Harry O'Flanagan and he made a really good job of it. He must be regarded as something of a pioneer in this polio work.

The End of a Hundred Year Epidemic

One of the most important things done in tuberculosis was to set up the National Report Centre. Some sort of feedback was essential to enable us to monitor what we were doing and how well we were doing it. So we established a Unit in Dublin Corporation Tuberculosis Department under Dr Gallen and organised it so that every new case of tuberculosis occurring in the country was reported to this Centre. Dr Gallen worked closely with Dr Michael Daly, who looked after TB on the medical side of the Department.

By 1958 I was coming home with Michael Daly, from some TB affair or other and I turned to him and said in a smug, pompous way, 'Do you know Michael, I am finally satisfied that we have a really first-class TB service.' He agreed, with equal self-satisfaction.

The next morning, he came into my office and said that Colm Gallen had been on the phone and that the number of new cases reported, which we knew to be dropping fast, had gone so far that for the previous month there had not been a single new case reported for the whole country. At the time, we really did not pay too much attention to this, feeling that it was a one-off occurrence. The following month, Dr Gallen came in himself to my office in the Custom House and told us that there had been no new case for the second month running. This in spite of the whole paraphenalia of mass radiography, the general practitioners, hospital outpatients, the lot all busy at work looking for cases. We sat there and looked at one another and I think I gave a kind of giggle. It took quite a while to sink in. Here was the tuberculosis epidemic, which had lasted for more than a hundred years and which had killed more than three-quarters of a million Irish men, women and children and on which we had been working for years, finally coming to an end. So far as I remember, we shook hands but otherwise were in a kind of daze. There were no victory celebrations or parades; I don't think we even went out for a drink to mark the event. We realised of course that the menace was still there and would return should we relax our defences.

A few years before, when we had presented the findings of the National Tuberculosis Survey to the Ulster Medical Society in Belfast and later to the British Tuberculosis Society at Edinburgh, there had been standing ovations. But a year after Colm Gallen coming in to give us the figures for the end of it, I was asked to read a paper on tuberculosis to the Statistical and Social Inquiry Society and so to speak wrap it up for good, and there were seven people there to hear the paper. People were bored with TB.

All over the world, the same thing happens; it happened in Britain over TB; when I went to Syria, even in districts where malaria had been rife, the only people who knew anything about it were the elderly — it was already forgotten; the same happened with yaws in Indonesia. Smallpox is already almost completely out of the public memory.

General Practitioner Research

In 1945, the Committee which produced the Plan for a National Health Service, recommended an enhanced and improved general practitioner service. In 1947, to do something about this, we began a national survey of the Dispensary System. This was aborted because of my departure from the Department at Dr Browne's invitation. In 1958 I made another attempt to start, when the dust had died down after the Mother and Child row. One of the features I wanted to see in an improved General Practitioner service, was a Research and Development unit. I had an especial interest in this, one because I had been myself a general practitioner who had carried out research and two, because I was in contact with different General Practitioner groups who were interested in doing some research and was in sympathy with their aims. The foundation of the College of General Practitioners made this even more practicable. What business of a size comparable with that of the General Practitioner Service, with the costs, with the aims, the problems and so on, could exist, much less prosper, without a Research and Development Unit?

There are academic departments of general practice, there

may be a research and development unit in the Department
of Health but for the ordinary front-line general practitioner
working with the people, they seem to me to be remote. I
came to the conclusion that I should restart the Dispensary
Survey again. We had already gone a very long way in developing the specialist services as outlined in the 1945 Plan, the
hospital building programme was going well but we needed
the scientific data to enable us to plan anything further. I
had several discussions with Mr MacEntee and tried to interest
him in the protection of vulnerable groups like students. They
needed special care, because they were at a growth period of
their lives, were under stress, many were away from home for
the first time and many suffered from neglect perhaps from
insufficient or the wrong kind of food, and many had nervous
problems due to inadequate funds or over-work or whatever.
These things laid the foundation for later ill-health. The later
illness caused by present-day neglect would be far more costly
to the country than any care given now.

I also talked about the aged, because people were living
longer and were likely to present a growing problem in the
future. We had to start thinking about their care now. I wanted
to make the care given by the general practitioner much more
preventive as well as curative as regards the people for whom
he was responsible. The mental health service particularly
needed reform as it was based too much, almost exclusively
on the asylums and we needed to take into account things
like stress and to involve general practitioners more in mental
health, the neuroses and the psychoses. I wanted in addition
to re-start the Dispensary Survey or general practitioner study
as well as to set up a 'health practice district' using County
Kilkenny as a suitable area. Mr MacEntee's response was
that the Cabinet were very well satisfied with what had been
achieved in the field of health. This was not the time to spend
money. He felt that I should relax, sit back and really spend
my time in 'polishing the machine'.

So I felt, rather sadly, that the great days of public health in
Ireland were coming to an end. I had been exposed in the East
to the poverty and health needs there, to such an extent that
I could not rest easy. So I wrote to Dr Candau and reminded
him that when in Ireland he had asked me to come to work

for the WHO. I told him that I was now ready to go for a longer assignment provided of course that he still wanted me. He replied that he felt that I should gain more experience in the Third World and that I would be hearing from Dr Mani, the Regional Director for South East Asia. Mani followed this up with an offer to me to become WHO Representative and Chief of Mission to Indonesia for two years. Mr MacEntee gave me leave of absence and I was processed and seconded to WHO. So with a small suitcase and a bag of books, I started off on my next adventure.

11

Indonesia

I WENT through the usual induction and briefing in Geneva. By this time I was used to it, but as this was a longer-lasting and more significant post, I spent a week studying the health and social conditions of Indonesia. Then I was sent on to New Delhi. Once again I was received by friends and quickly began to feel one of the team.

The Area Representative in Indonesia was in charge of the WHO team, numbering about 30 international people. His job was to look after them and to negotiate with the government on WHO Aid Programmes. But WHO was also going to appoint an Adviser in Public Health and also an Adviser on TB in Indonesia. I told Dr Mani, the Regional Director, that I did not want to be merely a travel agent or a diplomat, which the job implied. I had been Chief Medical Adviser to a country for years, also a consultant to WHO on TB and I would either do all three jobs or else the public health or TB jobs separately.

I had been tipped off on this by Ronald Bland, a Dublin man, a TCD graduate and a Fellow of the Royal College of Physicians of Ireland. He had started as a Medical Missionary in the Sudan and eventually through a senior post in the Sudan Medical Service, one of the best of the British Colonial Medical Services, he came to WHO in New Delhi, and was an outstanding person.

Bland advised me that where there was an Area Representative and a public health adviser, they always clashed. Dr Mani had had difficulties with this before and regarded it as something forced on him by Geneva. However, he agreed to give the idea a try on an experimental basis and to let me look after the three functions.

At the Indonesian embassy in Delhi I became good friends with Mrs Subandrio, the wife of the Foreign Minister and

Vice-President of Indonesia, who in her own right was the Vice-Minister of Health. She was the daughter of a former Regent of a district in East Java, a native ruler under the Dutch regime. Her husband, a good surgeon, had been pulled out of his practice in Semarang, a seaport town on the North Java coast, by President Soekarno. He was sent to London as Ambassador, then to Moscow, before being brought home and made Foreign Minister. Indonesia, in contrast to most Muslim countries, is noted for its redoubtable women. Although tiny and fragile and exquisite, they exercise enormous power and indeed in much of Sumatra there is a matriarchal society. Most of the women who had received a higher education during the time of the Dutch rule were aristocrats, the daughters of native rulers and were accustomed to giving orders and to be obeyed. The Ministry of Health also had Dr July Sulianti, who was a most important public health officer. The Chief of the Dental Service was also a lady.

The Dutch, who had held the Indonesian Archipelago as their East Indian Empire, for more than 300 years, had set up a magnificent Colonial Medical Service. But they never allowed the Indonesians to progress past the lowest level of medical qualification and when they left there were only 400 medical people so qualified to look after a population which at that time amounted to at least 80 million people.

In 1958, Indonesia was the sixth most populous country in the world. It stretched from the tip of Malaysia in a great crescent of islands down to near the north coast of Australia, about 3,000 miles and including 5,000 inhabited islands. Kalimantan, or Borneo, is a vast island as large as Europe and is called the 'green desert' since it is empty of people. Java on the other hand is one of the most densely populated places on earth. Indonesia has more than two hundred ethnic groups, and more than two hundred languages and was first Animist, then Buddhist, then Hindu, and is now Muslim with a few Christians here and there.

It has an ancient culture and was once a great Hindu empire. After three hundred years of colonial occupation by the Dutch, in a bloody war Indonesia secured its independence. The country was, in my time, a democracy of a sort, based on the Pantjasilas, the Five Principles. These were belief in one God,

Humanism, Nationalism, Democracy and Social Justice. There was complete religious toleration with an over-riding mild Muslim belief as the religion of the majority.

President Soekarno, the father of his country, had created a unified state, introduced a single language, and from 1948 had started to develop Indonesia as a world power. He aspired to become the leader of the Third World and of the non-aligned states.

Soekarno walked a tight-rope. He was balanced politically between an all-powerful army (a state within a state) and the PKI, the Parti Kommunisti Indonesia, an almost equally strong force. He ruled through a small devoted following of people like the Subandrios, but when the inevitable conflict occurred between the two great forces, he was shown to be a 'paper tiger'. The small following of Soekarno's, in between the military who had some Cabinet posts and the Communists who also had a few Ministers, were the people with whom I had to work.

My office was on a beautiful tree-lined avenue, near the centre of the city and just opposite the residence of the Commander-in-Chief of the army. I had an Indian barrister, Mr Bhatia, as WHO secretary, an Indonesian clerk-typist and a driver-messenger, but without any formal transport. I solved this by borrowing a jeep from the malaria crowd and settled in to deal with the other problems.

First, there was terrible poverty everywhere. Second, the country could not get up off its knees, because every viable industry was operated by army officers, with all proceeds going into the coffers of the armed forces.

So far as health was concerned, there was widespread malaria, tuberculosis, typhoid, an el tor cholera, serious malnutrition and worm infestation of children, inadequate water supplies of villages, serious infant mortality and, in Java, massive over-population. The Ministry of Health was grappling as best they could with these problems. Their staff on the technical side were first-class, honest, hard-working men and women. Due to inflation they could not live on their pay and were forced to carry on private practice from their homes at night. In any case the shortage of doctors was so great that the country could not afford that any doctor did not work all out.

The clerical workers were only good for a couple of hours work a day due to under-feeding. Owing to the frequent rebellions, the Ministry of Health was starved of day-to-day information on what was happening in large parts of the country and this was made worse by the island geography and the lack of regular, well-organised communications. The professional staff were so thin on the ground that the organisation was coming near to breaking point. The hospitals, apart from those run by missionaries, were inadequate and medical supplies just weren't there, nor had they the money to buy them abroad. On the other hand, the medical schools were beginning to turn out graduates of good quality in fairly large numbers, other training programmes were producing nurses and particularly a type of health administrator with a technical sanitary training and these were very good. For the first time there were a large number of bright youngsters who had had a good secondary school education and were available for further education. Then there was also the factor that people had become very 'health conscious' because of President Soekarno's propaganda and so were most cooperative.

Faced with such a situation, where did someone like me, coming fresh to this job, begin? WHO had a series of programmes and projects working with the government. When I had had a look at them, I found that a few were excellent and the rest limping along.

For example, Indonesia had a very large Yaws problem. We have never seen anything like it in Europe or America. A village might become infected and in a relatively short time everyone would develop great strawberry-type open sores, particularly on the arms and legs. If they were sufficiently severe or lasted long enough these could end up in great ulcers and bony deformities. With these things people just sat around and were miserable and of course no one could work, particularly in rice paddies. A village or kampong which does not grow sufficient rice, just does not eat. So apart from the pain and suffering, there was hunger as well.

Penicillin cures yaws, so WHO organised a great Yaws Eradication Programme for Indonesia. The work was carried out by the Indonesians themselves, using penicillin supplied by the United States. The work was organised in the first instance by WHO and then directed behind the scenes by us. Our role was to play it quietly. It was a complete success and I arrived just as it was really well under way.

To see an Indonesian village complex suffering from yaws was terrible. You could 'smell' a sick village or kampong. Ordinarily an Indonesian village had a sharp, spicy smell, with a small amount of the tropical 'must' but sharp and clean. The pace at which people moved about and the general atmosphere was clearly healthy. It is the intuition of the professional, just as an Irish cattle dealer can look at twenty animals in a field and tell you their weight dead-on to a few pounds.

But, to see a yaws health team arrive, do a census of the kampong, inject everyone with a shot of penicillin and then to come back three weeks later and find 90 per cent of the people's sores healed or nearly healed was little short of a miracle. Then come back three weeks later and give a second shot to anyone not healed up and to know that they too would be cleared in a few days was very, very satisfying. To see this carried out in village after village with the same results made you really believe in the magic of organised medicine.

It had a spin-off in that the ordinary people in the kampongs saw the benefit of public health and thereafter were only too anxious to cooperate and were friendly to foreigners like me moving amongst them. The real heroes of the yaws operation were the Indonesians themselves who did all the work.

We had begun a malaria eradication programme and this also was a huge undertaking. It was based on the following strategy. A person can be bitten any number of times by anopheles mosquitoes and nothing happens except a local irritation and annoyance. But if a mosquito has recently bitten and sucked up the blood of a person suffering from malaria and then bites you, it will infect you and you will develop malaria.

Years before Dr Pampano, the Director of Malaria at WHO Headquarters in Geneva thought up a plan based on the fact that once a female mosquito has had its feed of blood, it alights somewhere, usually on a nearby wall, to digest it. He concluded that if it were possible to spray the walls of houses with DDT, then when the mosquito, particularly the female, landed to digest the blood-meal, it would be killed. This would interrupt the transmission of the disease. It was obvious that it was not necessary to kill all mosquitoes but only those carrying the infected blood from humans.

But to spray all the houses occupied by 80 million people living in 5,000 inhabited islands and to respray them several times a year for a number of years was a gigantic task. But malaria was so bad in Indonesia that it was preventing all development so not to attempt this task was unthinkable.

At the ground level, it was a very simple operation, but the supervision necessary to ensure that it was properly carried out and that the correct amount of DDT was deposited on the walls and that no house was missed, was difficult. The logistics of maintaining supplies of DDT, spray guns and the recruitment, equipping, feeding and paying of staff was great. Then there was the task of training staff, of research and evaluation of results, all of which required special attention. Finally, there was the task of finding and recording cases of malaria, which became of importance as the campaign went on and the maintenance phase was reached. As the operation developed we were employing up to 15,000 spraymen and using up to two tons of DDT a day.

In addition to yaws and malaria there were two other problems in the communicable disease field. WHO had a pilot scheme for tuberculosis going on in Bandung, the great industrial centre of Java. It had been running for some years. I went to see it and found that they had done a good job under difficulties but that it had become static. Using their materials, I analysed their results and in a kind of round table approach came up with an improved development programme.

Leprosy was rife in Indonesia, and we had a very good French leprologist, Michel Blanc. One night talking about the spread of leprosy, he told me that he was seeing a 'cluster' effect. I got excited about this because what he described to me was the sort of thing I had seen originally in TB in Lurgan. He came up with a case-finding technique based on the 'clustering' idea. At first some of the WHO leprosy pundits did not accept this. However, Ronald Bland in New Delhi supported him and of course I was convinced that he was right. Michel's new technique meant that by examining people in close contact with known existing cases, you would find something like

90 per cent of all undiscovered cases. Instead of examining everyone in a kampong, you only had to check a few, but it was essential that you got this few, since they included all the undiscovered cases. This reduced the work and particularly the cost of case finding.

Lack of information was a problem in the Ministry. An epidemic of smallpox or el tor cholera could smoulder along for months on some remote island and the Ministry in Jakarta would know nothing about it. Suddenly it might burst out from the island and spread like wild-fire from one island to another and become difficult to contain. I found that the Americans working with the Indonesian police had developed a network of short wave radio stations, giving good coverage of the total country. Each day each station came in with information to police headquarters at Jakarta. With a bit of finagling and the help of good friends I got them to include health information with the police data, and this enabled me to set up a report centre in the Ministry.

This led to other things. For example, Java had 70 million people at that time and epidemic diseases were fairly well under control. But the introduction of some of the major epidemic diseases into Java would have been disastrous. Now all the major ports of Java were on the north coast. The idea was to stop the disease at these ports because there was a very large inter-island traffic. WHO had an English Port Sanitary Officer, Norrie Earthrowl, from Bristol to train a cadre of port sanitary officers to contain this problem. But to make sure, Dr Newell, our epidemiologist, organised the vaccination of all the people of the port areas of all the cities on the north coast of Java, from end to end, a magnificent job.

In clinical practice in Ireland, one could if one was lucky save the odd life. In the Custom House, there was the satisfaction in getting something started which, as in the case of tuberculosis, could lead to the saving of 4,000 lives a year. Equally, working for a reduction in infant mortality might help to bring it down by say 17 deaths per 1,000 live births and this meant that 1,000 babies each year continued to live. But in Indonesia these figures ran into hundreds and hundreds of thousands of people and one could see it happen. You yourself did not do it. In Ireland it was the medical and nursing cadres who did it, in Indonesia it was their poor underpaid, half-starved characters in their health services who were responsible, but you had a hand in it and the feeling was wonderful.

Our attack on malaria was not going well. It was mainly in the hands of elderly distinguished entomologists, nice old men, marvellous on mosquitoes but not very good at running an operation like this. As it was originally planned it was expected to end up as the biggest national health campaign ever to be staged in the world, but it had been badly planned and the execution was worse. When I first came to Indonesia I went to have a look at the Headquarters and to meet the staff. What I saw were broken-down jeeps, which had not been repaired for want of spare parts, poor storage facilities, which were important as even then we were using a ton of DDT a day and it was expensive, as well as other signs of bad management.

Then two things happened. First, when a new minister, an Army Brigadier, was appointed he happened to be a friend of mine so I brought him quietly to have a look at the place and recommended that he should bring in the Army to help. So he appointed a couple of well-trained, very active, young and intelligent army medical corps colonels to take charge. They brought with them a cadre of army medical personnel to stiffen the organisation. In a short time the operation was transformed. This did not mean that we no longer required the elderly malaria specialists. Their expertise was still required and they continued to be respected.

Soon after this operation, Dr Govindar Sambasivan arrived. Sam was a Brahmin from Kerala in South India. He had been a colonel in the Indian Medical Service, had a distinguished war record and served in Indonesia before. In the IMS he had become a very fine surgeon until he had taken up malaria and joined WHO. He was a small spare, abstemious man, a bachelor, a champion at tennis, full of fun and a great worker. We began a close friendship which lasted for 20 years till he died a year or so ago. Sam later came to Geneva, where he became Director of the Global Malaria Campaign. My wife and I were very devoted to him and he later came to stay with us in Rosslare.

Working closely with the Indonesian colonels, Sam put great heart into the campaign. It was replanned, starting with an 'attack' phase. This meant that the individual kampongs (or villages) and areas in towns were scheduled for attack. The types of mosquitoes found in the areas and their habitats were studied by entomologists. Houses were mapped, numbered and identified, even down to a hut on a paddy field. The houses were then sprayed. Spot-checks of spleen counts (people infected with malaria had enlarged spleens which could be felt on examination) and blood examinations, gave a base-line for the extent of malaria prevalent in a district.

Then followed a 'consolidation' phase. During this phase a regular spraying of houses at stated intervals took place and epidemics of malaria were monitored and controlled. Finally a 'maintenance' phase followed. For a certain length of time the population were under surveillance and a cadre of surveillants were available in the event of a recurrence of the disease anywhere. As a last part of the operation, a survey of an island, a province, or a country was carried out by a team of independent international surveyors, before certifying that the place was free from malaria. It was a vast and costly operation. In one way or another it involved the American 6th Fleet for logistics; the great oil companies; the UN Assembly; the US Senate; the US Congress; Soekarno; world medical, chemical, entomological research centres; WHO Headquarters at Geneva; UNICEF; the WHO Assembly at Geneva; the South-East Asia Regional Office at New Delhi; SEA Regional Meeting and dozens of other authorities, not forgetting the Indonesian Ministry of Health and the Indonesian Army.

The work was being done by the Indonesians. The USA supplied the DDT and the vehicles, which were an essential, with the Indonesians supplying the petrol. The US also supplied some equipment and in fact the bulk of the costs. UNICEF supplied the rest of the equipment including things like uniforms and footwear. WHO planned, supervised and executed and was the expert group in charge. The difficulties of the operation were very great since a slip-up anywhere, even when the disease seemed to be gone, could bring it back. If a government anywhere got fed up with the cost and dismantled the operation too soon, they had a recurrence. This happened in Sri Lanka and Syria and malaria did return. There was also the risk and indeed the certainty that mosquitoes might become resistant to DDT. WHO had a large organisation which coordinated chemical and biological research all over the world, stimulating, promoting and commissioning work in a rush to find alternative insecticides to DDT. My main role in this was to try to keep the train on the rails. For a month or two, I would not be needed and then some trouble would occur and within a day or so I was up to my neck in it. Then I was politely thanked and 'shooed' off again to the touch-line.

US Aid stretched in a long chain all the way back to Washington and was dominated by politics and technology. There was an annual vote in Congress on foreign aid and there was no certainty that any programme would be renewed. Then the Senate had a say in foreign affairs and their views carried weight. US politicians and officials might visit and had to be met. Depending on who they were or where they came from, the Minister and Sam trotted me out as Chief of Mission to meet some of them and with my red face, and an Irish accent and American links, I did my best to inspire confidence among the senators and congressmen in what we were doing. Our submissions for Aid had to be properly prepared and progress reports supplied, with annual reviews. I can confirm to the American taxpayers that their money was always well-minded and well spent.

Today, people regard this campaign in Indonesia and in other places as one of WHO's failures. But it really wasn't. To see what malaria was like before we started and to contrast it afterwards, showed that there was a tremendous improvement in the situation, even if it wasn't eradicated. Also everyone became educated in malaria, took their own precautions and the whole situation changed. I believe it would have succeeded only for the attempted coup by the PKI and the subsequent disturbances which set everything back. But the time, effort and money were not wasted.

Dyaks, Borneo

Meanwhile, I did studies on my own. After about six months in Indonesia I had become familiar with the problems of Java but I knew very little about things outside of Java. I was concerned about how to provide health services for the people on the smaller islands, what their health problems were and particularly what would be the logistics involved in a malaria campaign. So I went with a young American anthropologist up the Mahakam river in East Borneo and spent weeks in open boats, while I examined every man, woman and child in twenty dyak villages. At the first dyak village we came to, I saw outside one of the long houses a dozen or so peeled wands stuck in the ground. They were about four feet high and some at the top were carved to represent crude human figures. Others were cleft and carried an egg or a handful of rice wrapped up in a banana leaf. I was told that these were offerings to the spirits from someone who was ill. Being interested professionally, I went in to see further and found a poor wretch with ophthalmia in both eyes. This is a very severe infection of the total eye, rarely if ever seen today and usually means blindness, if the patient does not die from meningitis on the way. His two eyes were swollen up to the size of a bullock's and he was in dreadful pain. I went back to the boat, got some penicillin and gave him a huge shot. On our return down the river I went to see him and he had recovered completely. Since we were the first Europeans to go up that river for twenty years, the first to stop, the first to see his offering, the first with penicillin and so on, all the coincidences were sufficient to give that gentleman a firm belief in the power of his spirits.

Each village showed something interesting. In one they had a little old lady in a cage made from strong bamboo in a small hut. It seemed that she was an arsonist and they had caught her several times trying to burn down the Long House. The other old ladies came to visit and spend time with her, kept her in chat and brought her things to eat.

Apart from a great variety of fungal skin diseases and rashes and odd hernias and so on, they were an extraordinarily healthy lot. I could find no TB or yaws or really any public health problem. For example, I did not come across any heart conditions, raised blood pressures or chronic chest conditions even though they smoked a lot and our gifts of tobacco in each place were promptly grabbed by the Cephala Adat (headman). There was the odd badly-set fracture but most fractures seemed to have united well and cuts and wounds were not too scarred and had healed satisfactorily. There seemed to be more old people about than one would find in an Indonesian kampong.

I examined them all very thoroughly and they loved it. It

was interesting to see how many hernias there were among the men and they showed these to me very proudly. When I was examining such parts of their bodies, I noticed that most of the men had perforations across their penises. This had been described years before by Tom Hopkinson, who had seen it in the Sarawak Dyaks. Hopkinson said that they used to put chicken bones in the perforations to make intercourse more interesting. In a couple of the Long House apartments, I saw whitened chicken bones, hung up in looped affairs on the walls.

In one village the Cephala Adat was worried that they had had no children for some years. I was consulted and found that the average woman during her fertile period of life had up to thirty partners and the average man about twenty. The Cephala Adat blamed the women for staging some sort of sex strike. He talked vaguely about some sort of herb they had found in the forest.

In two or three villages, however, I did find bad outbreaks of malaria. In one Long House apartment after another, you could find whole families, lying in beds like boxes, covered with a bit of netting like a bit of old lace curtain to keep out the mosquitoes. They were shivering, sweating, pale and very sick. The whole Long Houses were more or less completely knocked out.

When I had done about twenty villages, I had seen enough. There was little abnormality to be found, but there was a problem with malaria. The exotic sex situation would have to await another day for someone else to deal with it.

Timor
Another of my expeditions was to Timor, at the far south-eastern end of the Indonesian Republic. One half of this great island belonged to Indonesia and the other to Portugal. The purpose of the visit, which was requested officially from New Delhi, was to see how we could organise yaws, TB and malaria on the island by coordinating the two services and administrations.

After a series of adventurous flights down the Sundanese Islands I got to Timor Koepang, the capital, where Dr Walther, an Austrian surgeon welcomed me. He was in charge of the local hospital, where I stayed. Timor Koepang was an interesting but violent place. Seventy per cent of all Walther's patients suffered from gun-shot wounds. Koepang had all the panoply of Indonesian government but their writ did not run outside the boundaries of the little city. The rest of the country was in the hands of the tribal chieftains, each with his own armed force. Once in a while they combined together and marched on Koepang, scaring the wits out of everybody, but always refrained from taking the place. Some of these chieftains were Catholic and some Protestants and now and again they had small religious wars, thus continuing the Thirty Years War after the Reformation, just as they do in Northern Ireland.

Dr Walther volunteered to drive me to Ocusi of Ambeno near the Portuguese border. The Indonesian authorities, who were supposed to help me, had been besieged by the chieftains recently and were too scared to stir out of the town. Walther and his head nurse, a very beautiful Chinese lady, whom he afterwards married and I, started off in his jeep to make the journey. From memory it was about 300 miles, but with Walther it was quite safe but sensational.

When I got there — to the Ocusi, the governor of Timor sent a plane to take me to Timor Deli, on the Portuguese side. For the first time in a hundred years or so, the town of Deli had had a face-lift and all the government apparatus had been cleaned up and painted. As part of this face-lift, the Portuguese Medical Research Council had sent out a team of good medical scientists to commence an examination of the tropical disease problems. The Portuguese Colonial Medical Service had not wanted it and the research team had been completely ignored. I insisted on the Chief Medical Officer coming with me when I went to see them, and it was the first time he had met any of them. The research team were very good technically and had good ideas for an excellent study of epidemic disease. But for some reason or other, and with the crowd in charge, nothing very much was likely to happen. Nor would any findings of theirs be implemented. This was the kind of stupid nonsense brought about through bad bureaucracy and mal-administration.

They had a poll tax, paid by the native population, who had to register themselves every year. I suggested that to make a start they should vaccinate everyone at that time, and since smallpox was endemic in Timor, they might begin this year. I also told them that I could get them the smallpox vaccine free from WHO. While they were at it, the research team could do a random sample check on the population to ascertain the problems they had to face. I offered to get someone from WHO to help them in this study.

The Indonesian part of Timor was just as hopeless, and, until the Indonesian army could establish some sort of order, or an arrangement could be come to with the chieftains, nothing was likely to happen. Later of course the Indonesian army took over the Portuguese end, which had been more or less abandoned by them. It has meant an era of bloodshed and there has been little peace on the island since.

The Karimunjawa Islands Survey
For some reason or other WHO found itself in possession of a small hoard of Norwegian kronors in 1958. Looking around for the best thing to spend it on, they decided to use it to have a small ship built which would serve the yaws campaign among the Indonesian islands. So the Norwegians went ahead and built a little beauty. It came out to Indonesia as a deck-cargo on an Italian liner. There was a 'handing-over' ceremony and a select band of Indonesian government notabilities and some WHO people had a day out, sailing around the harbour at Tandjongh Priok and up through the Pulau Seribu. But after that it lay for months in an isolated dock and I never could get them to use it.

At the request of the Ministry of Health I had been working on a health plan for Indonesia. Apart from the control or eradication of communicable diseases, the plan concentrated on providing simple medical care and particularly on the prevention of child deaths and the promotion of children's health so as to give them a decent start in life. With worm infestation, malnutrition and malaria, a tremendous number of children were anaemic, with pot-bellies and stunted growth. With protein deficiency a number were always on the verge of developing kwashiorkor. Every child had diaorrhoea several times a year during which time it was in negative nitrogen balance, which accounted for the stunted growth, failure to learn while at school and lessened resistance to disease.

Many countries faced with health problems like those in Indonesia developed their own methods of solving them. To provide ordinary or primary care the Soviets had the felshers or village doctors, the Chinese the barefoot doctors and so on. The Indonesians had a form of male nurse with a short clinical training in medicine and minor surgery. They were turning these people out in fair numbers and they provided simple care in the poorer districts of towns, kampongs and the islands. Some of these people became very good practitioners and it was a joke that one or two with large practices in Jakarta were employing fully qualified doctors as assistants. There is no way that you can stop the natural ability of such people; in the USSR a feldsher rose to become one of the greatest neuro-psychiatrists in the world and ended up as the Minister of Health of the USSR.

I decided to do a study to evaluate the services these nurses provided. I also wanted to see what supplements were needed to extend the range of care offered and how to improve the organisation. This was also linked with the use of the yaws boat and particularly on how to service medical care on the smaller islands.

So I organised a little expedition to the Karimunjawa Island archipelago of coral islands in the Java Sea. I invited some friends along to participate. We brought with us our servants and more important some malaria staff, some male nurses and four young Indonesian doctors. When we got to Tandjhong Priok, the harbour for Jakarta, we found half-a-dozen marines, with a couple of heavy machine guns and automatic rifles, to take care of us, as it seemed that the Karimunjawa Islands were 'bandit country'. There was also a truck with crates of Heineken beer and stacks of canned beef, courtesy of the Minister of Health and Mrs Subandrio.

Once we got to the islands our protocol was as follows. Each evening we would land on a different island. While films were shown* to attract the crowds and the nurses explained what we were about, a census was made of the population and each family was given a set of cards for the members. With the

*Courtesy of the US, borrowed for us by Barry Baûernschmidt who 'came along for the ride'.

young doctors, I went through the records of the island nurse for the previous year. I wanted to find out what kind of cases he had seen, what were his diagnoses, what treatment he had given and so on.

Then, starting at 5 am the next morning we put the entire population through a health examination, more or less to screen them, and anything unusual was left for me to look at. During this screening they had a spleen examination for malaria, were examined for yaws, leprosy and skin diseases, a blood specimen was taken for malaria and they were vaccinated for smallpox. Children were given BCG. As each test was done it was marked off on the person's card. The examination was usually carried out in the village school. People came in at one end and went along a line. As they emerged at the other end of the line and came out of the school, the village police-man checked the card to ensure that no one was missing out on anything. If anything was not recorded they were sent in again. We had had a search party under the village headman and anyone not attending was rounded up and brought in. People who were sick in their homes were visited. It sounds terrible, but it was all done with laughs and humour and for a community living on a remote island, a visit from a circus such as ours was amusing.

For us it was hard work; some days we saw seven hundred people. Then we packed up and went on to the next island and repeated the performance. Every five days we went back to base, analysed the results and compared what we had found with what the local nurse had found or treated during the previous year, and planned the next week's work. We finished the whole project in three weeks.

What we found was this. The nurses were highly competent and diagnosed and treated correctly the vast majority of illnesses. Their treatment was quite adequate, except that supplies of medicines might run out. They were not able to vaccinate for smallpox or give BCG to children. They did miss the odd TB case. Things like fractures were not so good and tumours requiring surgery remained untreated. We found bone deformities which could be corrected.

By regular visits from a ship like ours we could maintain medical supplies and provide for medical supervision and consultation for anything out of the ordinary and to take off cases needing cold surgery. I envisaged that we could use short-wave radio and later a flying doctor service. But our survey took place 30 years ago in revolutionary and dangerous times in Indonesia and when the place was 'broke'.

One thing in particular remains in my memory from this study. It was the discovery of a 'sick island'. When we got to this remote island, which did not have a nurse, there was a death-like stillness; no one came down to the shore to greet us and when we landed and walked up to the village we saw no one. Then we found that all the people were ill and lying in their houses.

There were two epidemics going on, one of yaws and one of malaria. The school was closed since all the children had died. People who could still stand were tottering about in their homes and they had not the wit or ability to go for help. They were hungry and helpless and had more or less given themselves up to die. It was pitiable. Fortunately we had enough penicillin to treat the yaws and then sent the boat back for food and for medicine for the malaria. When we had treated everybody, we left a nurse and some helpers to look after them. It was a lesson on what could happen to people on a remote island without communication.

As part of the job, I used to drop in on clinics and medical centres to see how things were going on, to study how they were operating the various schemes and to learn. One day I called at the main BCG Centre in Jakarta but found no one there. Hearing a noise, I opened a door and going in found all the girls of the BCG teams of Jakarta and the medical staffs, sitting about watching a film of President Soekarno's visit to America. They made me welcome and I sat down to watch it too. Later I asked the Director why they were not working. He said that they had not had any pay for two months, that the nurses, nice girls, were too tired and too hungry to go out and that in any case that they had no petrol. This last in a country which had more oil than they knew what to do with. So to cheer themselves up and till the money came through and they could eat again, they met every morning and had a film show. Things were like that in the cities, but in the country, the people in the kampongs could carry on.

My two years in Indonesia, from 1958 to 1960, were wonderful; there was always something new to get your teeth into, something to get started, always improvising, adapting, persuading, writing their new health service plan and many other ploys. At the end of my tour the regional WHO Conference of the South East Asian countries was to be held in the autumn of 1960 in Bandung. The Indonesians were anxious to act as hosts for this as they now had something to show and were proud of their progress. In addition they wanted to open their new Ministry of Health. My time was nearing its end and I had decided not to renew my contract in spite of Dr Mani's persuasion. My final contribution was to help them to prepare for the WHO Conference.

At the final meeting, on the last night of the Conference, which was also my last night, the Minister made a speech, thanking me for my work. This was followed by others and even by Ministers of Health from other countries and I thought it would never stop. When it came to my reply, I became so emotional that I could not finish, because I loved that country and its people. When I arrived home, they sent me a beautiful carved Balinese screen with a silver inscription.

Even more important, the Subandrios sent me their only child, Budoyo, to educate in Ireland. I put him in Clongowes, where my son James took care of him. Afterwards he studied economics at University College, Dublin where he got a good degree. Budoyo was a fine young man, became his father's assistant, then the editor of a journal, but later was directly or indirectly a victim of the tragedy of Indonesia.

The day after my return home, I went into the Custom House and to my old office. Walking into the room I found Charlie Lysaght sitting in the chair. He got up at once and came around the desk, took me by the hand and put me in the chair and said 'Sit down there. Thank God you are back safe and well, and now for heaven's sake stay there'. So I was back where I started, having had my fun, never more to roam.

It was most pleasant to take things up again and to go on as before. A great deal had been done in my two years or so of absence, death rates had continued to fall, hospitals to be built and the place was going on well. I decided to restrain myself in the future, to run around less and not to provoke people. In the Department the emphasis had come to centre

more and more on the administrative side, but the old programme was being followed and progress was being made. We
had a good service now, run by good people and one could
sit back. But every now and then would be a picture in my
mind of the homeless children of Calcutta, living in doorways
and hungry, or conditions in the shanty kampongs of Jakarta,
the poverty in the slums of Colombo or the sad harshness of
Somali life. One did not rest easy.

Then it started again. In 1961, WHO called me to Geneva
to become a member of a World Expert Committee on Dental
Education, about which I knew nothing. I was the only medical
person on the Committee, amongst a lot of world-famous
Dental deans and heads of Schools of Dentistry and Chiefs of
International Dental Organisations, a cross section of world
dental leaders. The WHO people explained to me that whenever
these great men soared up into the exotic realms of higher
dental thought, I was to pull them down to earth again as a
good public health man. I was to ask them how they proposed
to turn out more dentists to meet the ordinary needs of populations; how to introduce more of the preventive side of dentistry, and how to extend services and stop dentistry becoming
in many countries, any further, a money-making elite. I was
to insist on getting answers.

From the point of view of my distinguished and really
wonderful colleagues on the Committee, I was a nuisance. I
was also most irreverent, because when they got uppity on
the subject of what was really a dental monopoly, I kept taunt-
ing them with the magnificent work I had seen done by Chinese
quacks on the Dyaks. Actually it was not fair, but that lot
needed it. By digging my heels in, I helped to produce a good
Report which had a wide influence. I did not write the Report,
it was my colleagues but I asked the questions and made them
provide the answers.

It seemed to have worked for me, as I was asked back again,
this time to consider the training of Dental Nurses and Auxili-
aries. This was also of interest and I met the same kind of
dental authorities and really came to enjoy them as they were
first-class people. I seem to remember being also on some kind
of Committee on Public Health Administration in Geneva
and on the International Expert Panel of Public Health Administration, where I was a member for eighteen years.

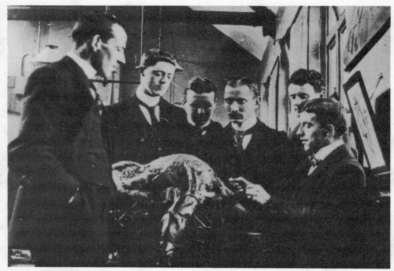

1899. An historic medical photograph. My father, Michael Deeny FRCSI, as Pro-Sector giving an anatomical demonstration in the Dissecting-Room of the Catholic Medical School in Cecilia St in Dublin. Left to Right, Kieran Fleury (Later GP, Birr), James Meenan (Later Prof Medicine UCD), T.T. O'Farrell (Later Prof Pathology UCD), Maurice Hayes (Later Prof Materia Medica UCD) and A.N. Other.

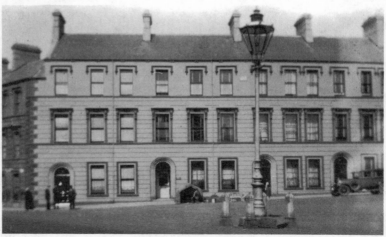

1927. Church Place, Lurgan where the story began. Taken at 11.10 am Tuesday 19 July 1927. The end house had a moment of fame in 1943-44 when it was the residence and Hqrs Mess of General Collins, who commanded the US Fifth Army, the first American troops to come to Europe during the Second World War.

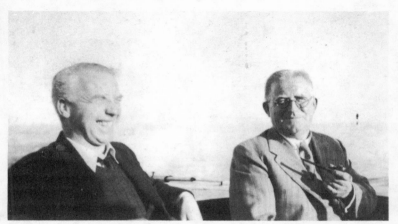

1937. Partners. My Father and I fishing in the Irish Sea, off Greenore, Co. Louth.

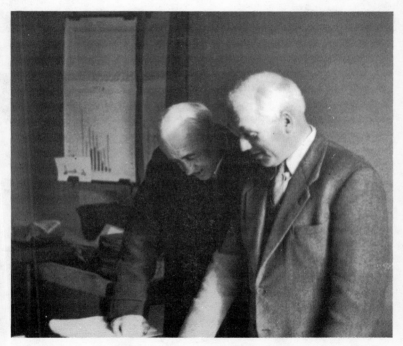

1954. J.D. MacCormack and myself in the office in the Custom House Dublin.

TELEPHONE
BELFAST 22859

AREA SECRETARY
S. KYLE

AMALGAMATED
TRANSPORT & GENERAL WORKERS UNION

REGISTERED OFFICES.
Transport House.
SMITH SQUARE. WESTMINSTER. LONDON. S.W.1.

AREA No. II

DISTRICT OFFICE
66, VICTORIA STREET,
BELFAST.

GENERAL SECRETARY, ERNEST BEVIN
ASSISTANT GEN. SEC. ARTHUR DEAKIN.
FINANCIAL SECRETARY, STANLEY HIRST.

15th. June, 1940.

Dr. J. Deeney, M.D., M.Sc.,
Church Place,
Lurgan.

Dear Doctor Deeney,

At a meeting of our Textile Council held here in Belfast, I was directed to convey to you their sincere thanks and appreciation for the splendid work you have done, and are doing on behalf of Textile Workers in Lurgan, particularly , and the Textile Workers throughout Northern Ireland in general.

I brought to the notice of our Council your very excellent work, and they were delighted to know of your public-spitited action.

Yours is the first work of the kind to be carried out in a Technical and Scientific manner in the Textile Industry. The results so far reveal an appalling state of affairs.

At our conference with the Power Loom Manufacturers Association on 11/6/40, I quoted from both your Pamphlets to show the results accruing from low earnings. In all Wages Conferences your work is most useful. Again on 13/6/40, I quoted you at a meeting of the Rope, Twine & Net Trade Board, and the Chairman Mr. S. Reid, (a Solicitor) was so interested that he asked me whether I could provide him with a copy of both Pamphlets. If you could oblige I will have them passed along.

Perhaps I should state that our Textile Council consists of representatives of all sections of the Linen Trade in this Union in Northern Ireland and represents approximately 10,000 members.

In conclusion I should like to add my personal word of thanks for your splendid efforts on behalf of the worst paid Textile Workers in the British Isles, and to assure you that if I can assist in this worthy object in any way I am yours to command.

Yours faithfully,

District Organiser.

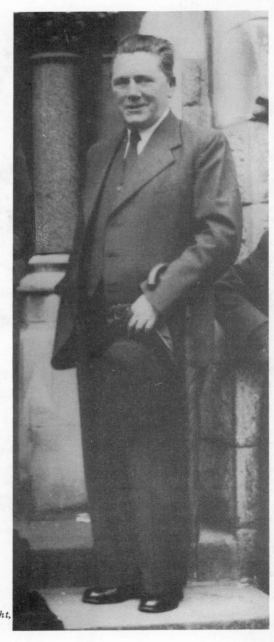

*1955. Dr Charles Lysaght,
CMO, my successor.*

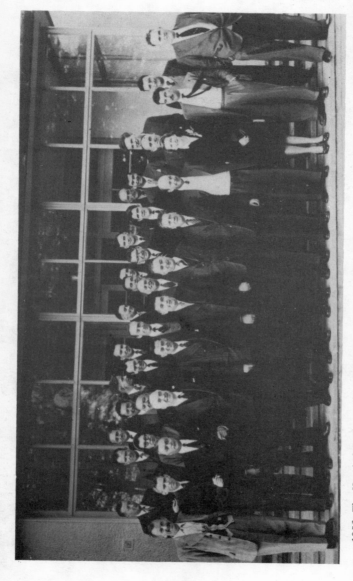

1956. The Hospital Builders. Group taken at the opening of St Stephen's Hospital, the Southern Regional Sanatorium, Cork. Front row, — — Flood (Engineer), Deeny (CMA), Norman White (Chief Architect), — Michael Jordan (Chief Engineer), Chas. Lysaght (D/CMA). Steve Cotterel and Brendan O'Herlihy are in the second row, behind Michael Jordan.

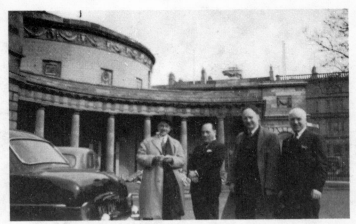

1957. Visit of Dr M.C. Candau, Director-General of the World Health Organisation. Group taken at the Rotunda. J.D. MacCormack, Candau, Tom Murphy and author.

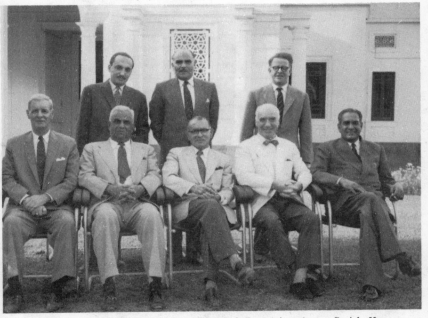

1958. WHO Area Representatives for South-East Asia, taken at Patiala House, New Delhi at the Regional Conference. Front. Dr Fitzmaurice (Can) Thailand, Gen. Puri (Ind) Burma, Dr Mani (Ind) Regional Director, Dr Deeny (Ire) Indonesia, Dr Tuli (Ind) Sri Lanka. Back. Dr Lucien Bernard (Fr) India and DHS, Dr Thant (Ind) Nepal, Dr Hewitt (Scots) Afghanistan.

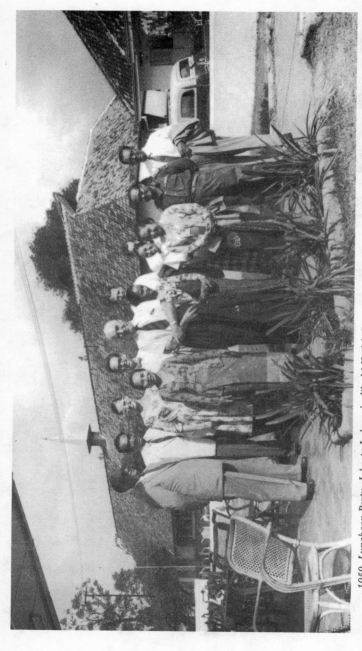

1959. Luncheon Party, Jakarta Indonesia, World Health Day, April 1959. Front, from left, Dr Ossorio-Tafall (UNDP Chief), Mrs Subandrio (V/Minister of Health), Deeny, Gen. Subarto (in uniform) (Minister of Health), Dr Dadi (Director of Health Services), Indonesia.

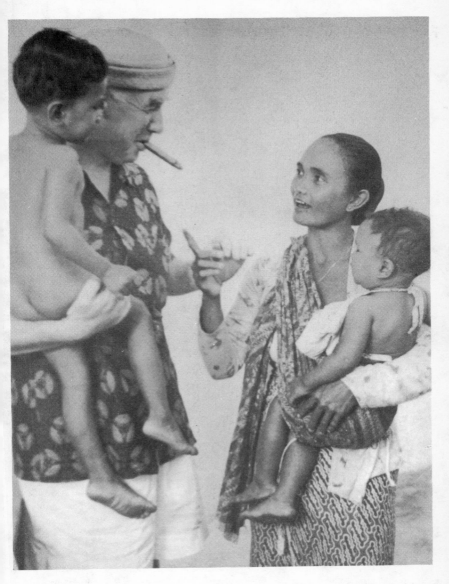

1959. Island Health Survey, Karimunjawa Islands, Java Sea. A Public Health discussion.

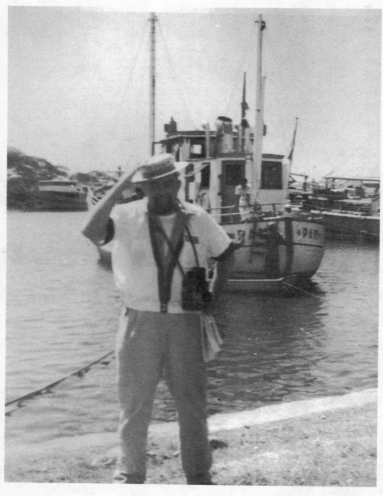

1959. Karimunjawa Islands Survey. Loading the *Pam*. Barry Bauernschmidt
— our wonderful American.

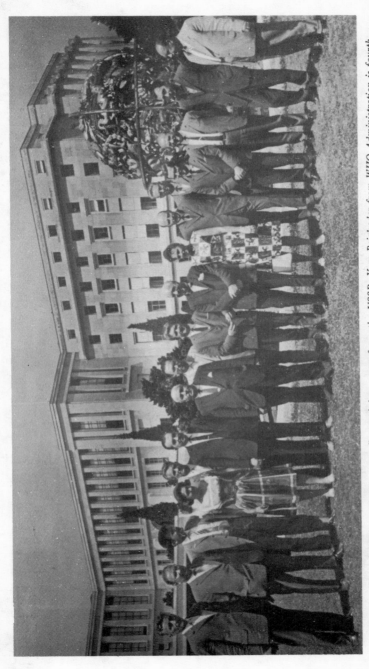

1962. Palais des Nations Geneva. My first training group from the USSR. Yves Beigbeder from WHO Administration is fourth from the right.

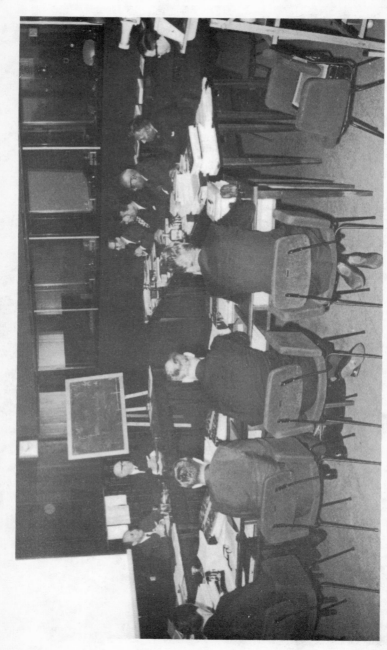

1964. World Health Building Geneva. Senior Staff Training. Dr Candau, DG addresses a Senior Training Group.

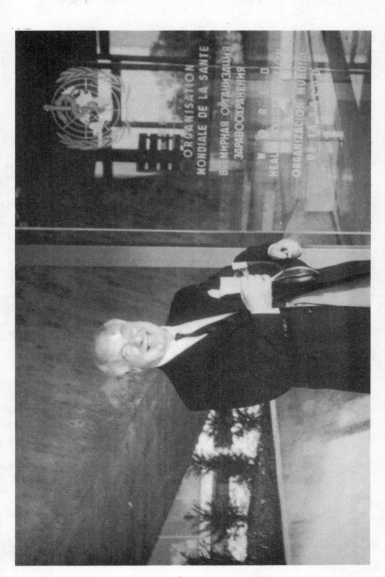

1967. Leaving WHO on my last day as Chief of Senior Staff Training, 1 Oct 1967.

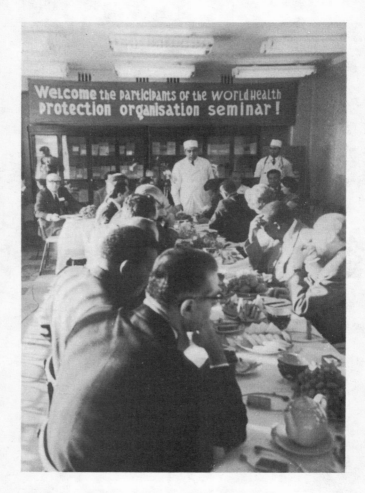

1969. Director, first WHO Travelling Seminar in USSR on Post-Graduate Medical Education. Reception and Address by Chief Surgeon, First Medical Institute, Moscow.

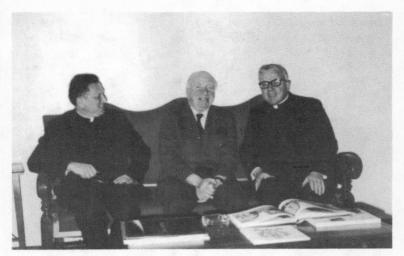

1970-71. The Secretariat of the Pontifical Council, Cor Unum, Vatican, Rome. From left Archbishop Kada, Deeny, P. de Riedmatten OP.

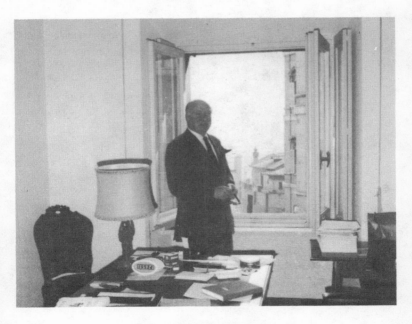

1970-71. My Office in the Vatican.

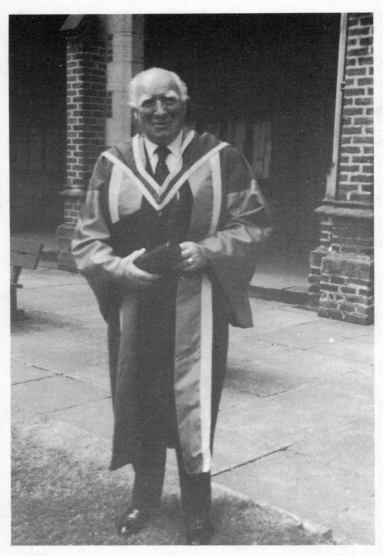

1983. Honorary Doctor of Science, Queen's University of Belfast. I put this one in because Public Health men and women being usually in the 'backroom', seldom receive such an honour and to show that it is appreciated.

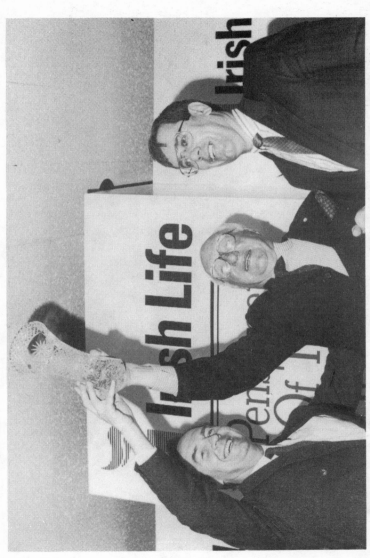

1988. Irish Life National Pensioner of the Year. From left, Dr Michael Woods, Minister for Social Welfare, the author and Brian Duncan, FIA, General Manager (Ireland) Irish Life Insurance Company.

12

WHO Training

IN THE spring of 1962, I was telephoned from Geneva and asked would I come for three months, to train the first group of people coming from the USSR to work for WHO. I was not particularly keen on this, especially because there was a strong political slant to it, and I had one son doing a PhD at an American university and a second likely to go. I did not want to queer the pitch for them. I went to see Mr MacEntee and told him about it. He said not to turn it down and the next morning sent for me and said that he had spoken to Mr Lemass, the then Taoiseach about it, who said 'it's an excellent thing that the Russians are coming to work for the UN at last and an honour that an Irishman should be asked to train them. Tell him to go!' So I went.

WHO recruited its own staff from all over the world. Anyone, anywhere in the world could apply to WHO for a post and if a post was vacant and they were the best qualified for the job, they were hired. Sometimes, as in my case, if they wanted you, they would start a kind of head-hunt. There was a two-way traffic. A certain amount of attention was paid to geographical distribution of staff so that the organisation did not become a European or American preserve. Of course a constant stream of ambassadors called to 'present' people on behalf of their governments, usually minister's friends or politician's sons, but they never got anywhere and WHO reserved the right to appoint whoever they wanted. The USSR, though participating in the Assembly and contributing to the funds, in fact being the second largest contributor, had never had any of its nationals employed, except for an Assistant Director General and one senior cancer expert.

Then in 1962, out of the blue, the government of the USSR wrote saying that they were sending some people along and would WHO please employ them, or words to that effect. This created a problem as no government was going to tell WHO who to employ. So there were negotiations and a compromise was reached. The USSR submitted several hundred of their best candidates for a range of posts and WHO sent a team of senior people to Moscow, authorised to select those whom they were prepared to consider for employment. It was this lot that I was to try to turn into international civil servants.

They arrived at Geneva on an Aeroflot plane and I met them at the airport. My first effort was to introduce myself and to give each of them 100 Swiss francs, as we felt that they might not have been allowed to take any money out of the USSR. They were fixed up with an hotel and some folk from the Russian Embassy took charge of them for the night. They were mainly young and yet distinguished bio-medical scientists, most of whom had never been out of the USSR before. They were home-sick and scared, and came with only the clothes they wore.

I met them formally the next morning and they were very deferential, calling me Professor, which I was not, but I impressed them a bit by asking them to call me Academician, which I was, as a Member of the Royal Irish Academy and which really 'ranked' with Soviet people. We went on a walk-about in Geneva and when they saw the wealth of the Swiss, they had a cultural shock. This was only the beginning, since I wanted them to understand that in their international work they would see a range from riches to extremes of poverty, neither of which they had ever experienced in the USSR. As they had only a few words of English or French amongst the group of more than twenty persons, we started with good interpreters.

As we sorted one another out, it was plain that they were an interesting lot. I took to them from the start. They hadn't a clue as to what WHO was or what it did. The gap between their lives and understanding and anyone else's outside of the Iron Curtain, was unbelievable. I commenced them on English language study and was surprised to find that they had been studying without effect for months in English and French language schools run by the Ministry of Health of the USSR in Moscow and Leningrad.

It was interesting to see how the cultures clashed. For example, it took weeks for them to understand what an administrator was. In the USSR, the entire health organisation, financial, scientific, legal, planning the lot was run by technically qualified people. The British-Irish concept of the lay official or administrator puzzled them. They could not understand how anyone could claim to have knowledge or ability to do anything without proper technical training. When I brought WHO people along to talk to them, they usually began by describing WHO's policy towards this problem or that situation. After a bit, my Russians said 'Please, no more policy, what does WHO actually do?'

My job was to broaden them out to mix and work internationally, to reduce their suspicions and to get them to change, without feeling that they were letting the side down or betraying their principles. After a bit, I found the magic formula which brought us all together. We were all doctors, doing the job that doctors do all over the world. We respected one another as doctors and had a common interest as doctors, which transcended ideology, nationality, race, colour, culture or anything else. It was also important to impress this approach on my colleagues in WHO who met them.

When I had them fairly well on, I found that no one in the organisation wanted to employ them. Jobs for which they were well suited suddenly disappeared. People were afraid of them. Now you cannot have a real international organisation unless you have everyone working in it together. So with the Director-General's agreement, I went around 'placing' them, and where I met opposition, I called on him to use his 'big stick'. I had trouble from the other side as well, one day two fellows from the USSR embassy accused me of 'needling' them on ideology. I threw them out politely and said the people were now working for WHO, and if they did not like it they could take them home. I did eventually get them settled into jobs, but not really as good as they were worth.

Of course the group soon knew what was going on and before they left for their assignments, they gave a most expensive dinner party in the most expensive hotel in Geneva for my wife and I. Much to her amusement, I was given a hug and a Khrushchev kiss by every one of them. The whole thing became something of a joke among my friends and throughout the Palais des Nations I came to be known as 'The Father of the Russians'. When the job was done and before leaving for home, I asked Dr Candau why he had picked me for this task and he said 'we thought that only an Irish Catholic policeman could handle it'.

WHO Senior Staff Training

After the first training course for USSR nationals, and then the Dental Expert Committee on the training of dental nurses, I was asked to remain behind after the meeting. They said they wished to discuss the setting up of a WHO Staff College; in fact shortly after we had commenced, they asked me would I undertake to start it. They had been impressed with the job done on the group of USSR people and felt that I could take it on. They said that there was very little money for it and it was obvious that they had really very little idea as to what form it should take. The overall responsibility for the operation was to rest with Dr Fred Grundy, Assistant Director General, of whom more hereafter.

It was apparent that WHO was taking a chance both on this project and in selecting me to start it. I came home to Dublin and resigned from the Department of Health in October 1962 and made it back to Geneva. I could have asked for further leave of absence, which might have been granted, but my friends and colleagues had loyally kept my place to return to, and it was only fair to them to give it up.

WHO had been started by hard, tough, magnificent but compassionate men and women. They had mainly come from former colonial health services or post-war aid programmes, were austere and dedicated and technically were competent. The organisation was run on a shoe-string and there was no waste of men or money, and they had passed this tradition on. It was now staffed by a much more varied lot, most of whom had come up through national health services, research institutes or were specialists in fields like tuberculosis who had broadened out into public health and had become high-level 'generalists'. They were growing older and would have to be replaced. I had to think about what work WHO would do in the future and what kind of people with what skills and knowledge would we need to do it. The future of WHO would depend on these people and what we made of them.

There were no guidelines and no real money and no staff. There was also the problem that WHO had no premises of its own. We were lodgers in the Palais des Nation, which was owned and administered by the UN proper. We were tucked in here and there in odd corners and it was clear that there was no room there for the Staff College.

The structure of WHO was based on the concept that people would come from international organisations, national health services, universities or research institutes from all over the world, would work and contribute and then after a period return home. You were appointed for a five year period on contract, the first two being probationary, were given a defined field or assignment and then it was up to you to produce. If you did not produce, then you went home. It was tough on staff but very good for WHO. If you produced and went on producing, then they kept you on. WHO had over the years developed a hard core of people of proven reliability, integrity and dedication, who really made the organisation move. These were usually high-level 'generalists', possibly specialists who had broadened out. Others were public health men and women who had come up due to their ability, often from low level posts and with increasing responsibility to senior positions in national health services.

As a world organisation WHO had people stationed in countries all over the world. Such people could become isolated and could lose touch with world programmes. As a fact of life, the better a man or woman did their job, the more likely he or she would be left there to do it. Their immediate superiors would not want the trouble of any disturbance or of replacing them. Of course this was the kind of person we wished to reach with our training.

While I had little or no money, I had immense resources. In fact I had a ready-made faculty, in that WHO in Geneva had the greatest single collection of medical expertise in the world in relation to the fields in which it was interested. In Western Europe, there were available experts in subjects which WHO could not cover. Properly handled they would feel privileged to be invited to teach, as our staff were an elite group working all over the world.

It was apparent that the Staff College, such as it was likely to be, should as a first priority provide for a flow of information, not only from the top downwards but from below to the top. A second priority was to ensure that courses of training would provide a constant review of WHO's methodologies and techniques by the discussions which would go on in the groups, by the people who carried out the operations in the field. A third priority was to balance the training groups by selecting people from different levels of the organisation, so that they should educate one another. A fourth priority was to supplement their professional knowledge; they should learn new techniques and be exposed to new ideas, whether in management, medicine, social psychology, operations research, the dynamics of change and other concepts such as systems analysis.

In addition to our own headquarters staff, expert in their respective fields, we had outside teachers. Howard Perlmutter from IMEDE in Lausanne taught social psychology; Professor Roget came from the University of Geneva to teach sociology as it might be applied to medical problems; Brian Abel-Smith from the London School of Economics taught social administration; Joe Logan, a good County Down man from Bangor, the Chief of the British Medical Research Council Unit in Manchester came to talk on the organisation of primary health care and was supported by Teddy Chester, the expert on social planning from Manchester University. We had management consultants from Paris and London; the officer in charge of Planning from the Surgeon-General's Office in Washington, Dr Kissick, was particularly appreciated.

I believed that it was not enough for scientists to be world-beaters in their field. It was also important that they should know something about management, how to run things and how to plan and organise change. After all, if they had the intelligence to become a good scientist they could also become good managers.

Overseeing the whole operation was Fred Grundy. The idea of a Staff College was largely his and in the working out of the concept he played a large role. Apart from the encouragement he gave me, he kept others from interfering, the people who wanted to climb on the band-wagon like all politicians or even to take over, when we had the thing going. He gave me a free hand but was always there to provide wise counsel. A good, solid, wise, sensible, decent Englishman, it was a pleasure to work with him.

I was blessed during my time by a succession of first-class secretaries: Adrienne Radbone, Desiree MacCready, Kathleen Hargreaves and Helen Legh-Jones. They minded me, took care of everything and neither time nor trouble prevented them from getting the work done in a superlative way. I even gave them away when they were married, and indeed the relationship was really one of a father and daughter.

One of the things that helped these courses was that people saw that those who attended them and who had been stuck in a job, began to move. At the end of each course, I prepared an assessment or evaluation on each participant for the Director-General. These were invaluable to him as these people counted in the future development of WHO and an independent judgement helped in fitting the right man to the right post. Of course he talked to many other people too. As well, I was given responsibility for the Fellowship Programmes for WHO staff and was able to link the course with a further period of study somewhere, say in a Research Institution to work out some research problem. Then the word got around that these courses were interesting and people from Headquarters, from Regional Offices, even new Regional Directors began to be included. Out of these training courses, as a result, to a greater or lesser extent of the dialogue between the top-brass of WHO and the groups which included so many with field experience, came various developments. For instance, the role of the WHO representative in countries was changed and they were given more power and scope. At the same time one was free to start things or to introduce new concepts in the working of WHO. For example, in 1963, I found that our statisticians, like most of that profession the world over at that time, were not a bit enthusiastic about computers and saw little need for them. So, as an experiment I set up a computer class at Headquarters and invited a mixture of some of the very bright people as well as the organisation's chiefs to attend. I was helped by Harry Whitfield, later to become Chief of Data

Processing in WHO. He was a great-hearted man who had been in the Department of Social Welfare in Dublin and was exactly suited for the job as he had a mind like a razor. We eventually put the entire senior staff of WHO through computer training.

Also in 1963 I did a study on audio-visual aids to teaching, partly from the point of view of our own training work and also from the point of WHO's role in education of all kinds. I got involved with language laboratories, teaching machines, techniques of planned programme instruction and all kinds of gadgets and gimmicks.

One of the things about WHO was that one was never idle. As a generalist public health man having, as I had, the odd slack time in between courses, they kept me busy. I was given the job of carrying out the study, ordered by the Executive Board, of evaluating WHO's services to countries and this took some time. Then I gave seminars in Dakar in Senegal for administrators from African countries, which had something to do with the Organisation of African Unity. I did the same thing in Amsterdam in the Dutch Overseas Institute and in other places and other countries.

I was sent to Gabon in West Africa as a Consultant on the organisation of a health service. Gabon was a former French colony, was originally established by the French as a haven for liberated slaves and is the richest single piece of the earth.

When I got there, which was during a revolution, I was taken on a tour of the country to see the health services by General Marcel Bonnaud, the WHO representative, and a French medical colonel. We had an old Dakota plane, seemingly one of the earlier models and showing it. In turbulence the wings went up and down like a seagull's. I was told that this was part of a local airline owned by some French film star. There was a elderly grizzled French pilot who drove the yoke with a Gaulois cigarette hanging out of a corner of his mouth. The inside was empty except for three little canvas seats. Within five minutes of take-off we entered a tremendous build-up of cumulus cloud. The pilot dodged and twisted and one minute it was pitch dark and the next minute the plane was flooded with blazing sunlight and was flung about like a falling leaf. Each time that we performed some particular aerobatic and the plane seemed to be about to fall to pieces, the pilot would turn, give a deprecatory wave of his hands and say, 'Pardon, mon general, pardon mon colonel', and then to me, 'Monsieur', light another Gaulois and carry on.

At Monila, in the interior, I saw something which shocked me. I was wandering about the hospital and came out of the back gate looking for a small leper colony, established by the Order of Malta which they had asked me to look at and report on. On a stone near this back gate, I saw a young woman seated with a child of about three years of age in her arms, the child was covered with confluent smallpox and was likely to die. Looking down, I saw that her left leg was swollen up with elephantiasis and that this vast lump she would carry with her till she died. Also, the foot seemed to be inflamed and possibly gangrenous. Hardened as I was, I felt pretty sick. To think that this was 1965 and with all the progress that science had made and that the situation was preventable, and to think further that this was what life had done to her and that it need not have happened, revolted me. She was waiting for admission, but what they could do for her or her child, I could not tell.

I went on and after a bit saw a flag flying with the Cross of Malta and eventually found a path in through the bushes into a compound where there was a collection of huts and a crowd of lepers sitting about. They were deformed and misshapen, but they chatted and laughed with me. They were well-fed and cared for and as happy as anyone could be under such circumstances. The treatment they were getting was fairly simple, but this was the same sort of thing as Dr Albert Schweitzer's world-famous colony not far away. But I could not get the picture of that poor woman and her child out of my mind.

In Libreville, the capital of Gabon, the French had built a magnificent hospital as part of the package they handed to each new government. The hospital was exactly the same sort of thing that you might see on the Riviera. Beautiful rooms for the top establishment and the Europeans, elegant semi-private accommodation for the middle-level civil service and the sergeant class and a good bit back, in the old hospital, the 'indigenes' lay in over-crowded squalor. The grounds, which at one time had been beautifully landscaped had become a shambles. The architects had either not known or ignored the fact that in West Africa each patient had his family and friends, who camped in the grounds while he or she was in hospital and cooked for the patient and themselves.

In the past, the highlight of the French colonial medical service was 'La Grande Endemie'. This was a very fine epidemic disease control system, common to all French colonies and I saw it at work just before it started on its way out. La Grande Endemie consisted of skilled native orderlies under the direction of a French medical officer, who visited rural areas. Each villager had a card and was legally obliged to turn up for examination, when the health caravan visited the village.

Everyone was examined for leprosy, sputum (if present) for TB, had a rough physical check-up and malaria blood-smears. But the thing that interested me most was that this was a 'sleeping sickness' area and they took specimens of spinal fluid. Now I remember the first time I tried my hand at lumbar puncture and introducing the six inch needle in the exact place in the spine at the exact angle, required terrific concentration. But these fellows sat down ten people on a bench, bent them over and one person nonchalantly popped in the needles in a sleight of hand movement and by the time he had in the tenth needle, the spinal fluid was flowing in the first. He strolled back to collect the samples and an assistant followed pulling out the needles. Sadly, this great work is coming to an end. With independence, the first thing people do is to tear up their cards, since it is no longer compulsory.

I went to see a kind of hostel place they had in the bush for sleeping sickness patients. Dozens and dozens of men and women lying around on mats in a deep sleep. Some could be awakened in a sort of way, but promptly went to sleep again, almost immediately. Most of them were in the prime of life but it was a living sleeping death.

France maintained about 1,500 army doctors in their former colonies and I visited some of them in the bush. We would be met at some meeting of trails by the officer, always wearing the plum-coloured kepi of the army medicals, always in a stiffly starched tropical uniform and on parade. They would salute: 'mon General, mon Colonel and Monsieur' and then we would follow them at high speed to their clinics or health centres or little hospitals. These were never up to very much, because France if generous in one sense, seemed to do things on a shoe-string.

After a while, the WHO Staff Training programme began to receive attention from outside. I had visits from, amongst others, officers of the Brookings Institute in the US and from the Rockefeller Foundation. The Carnegie Institute in Geneva laid on an international study on staff training and our programme was examined. The way we went about it became something of a main theme. Then in 1966, the American delegation to the WHO assembly asked for a discussion on our training system and asked too that I should make a presentation.

Dr Candau, the Director General, sent me on a mission to the Caribbean and several countries in Latin America to study with them and advise on their National Health Planning. I was also invited to Moscow and Leningrad as Consultant to the USSR. This last was particularly interesting as after a few days I had more or less the run of the Ministry of Health and it was interesting to see it in action.

WHO Staff Association

One day some members of the staff came to me and asked me would I become President of the Staff Association. This opened up a new activity for me, dealing with people and outside of my ordinary work and so I became a trade union official.

When WHO started in 1948 or so, a lot of the ideas of its structure came from the American civil service. In fact the first Assistant Director General, who looked after Administration and Finance, was an American, Milton P. Siegel. There was also an input of ideas from the British and French civil services and some of the practices were modelled on large US commercial undertakings.

The responsibilities and duties of each staff member were carefully defined, so that you knew where you were. On the other hand the staff member was protected by a set of rules, which amounted to a Bill of Rights. So between the staff member's responsibility to the organisation and the organisation's responsibility to the staff member, everything seemed to be covered. However, there were the odd grey areas. This is where the Staff Association came in. Each person's performance was evaluated each year by his or her superior officer and this was checked in turn by an officer superior again. It was shown to the staff member and one could appeal if there was dissatisfaction. Finally a person had a right of appeal through effective machinery right up to the UN Appeals Tribunal, where the case would be heard by a judge of international standing, such as Lord Justice Devlin. All this was necessary to ensure fairness, particularly with an organisation employing people from more than ninety nationalities and with infinite shades of culture, ideology and attitudes.

WHO was engaged in the construction of a new headquarters building at this time and the Staff Association was very much concerned with this. Such matters as accommodation for the staff enterprises, facilities for recreation, canteen and restaurant and other things were discussed. The Staff Association had all kinds of responsibilities ranging from the organisation of the Staff Ball during the Assembly week, children's parties, craft classes, art exhibitions and staff welfare generally, working closely with our welfare officer. There were interests like housing, working hours, casework of all kinds involving representation, communications like staff magazines, holiday centres, finance, etc. We had to deal with a constant stream of complaints, some trivial and some serious and all these had to be taken up and negotiated with administration.

We had a team of negotiators, who in a decent and honourable way, with forceful bargaining, could always secure a good result or a satisfactory compromise. Our success was due to always preparing our cases carefully. If the two sides to a dispute respect one another and are determined to seek a settlement, a fair solution can always be reached. A bad strike record or bad industrial relations are as much an indictment of inept or unjust personnel management as of bad trade union practice.

I kept WHO out of trouble, helped to improve conditions and helped to move us into the new building and to settle down. I was elected for a second term and was about to start a third when I suddenly felt that it was becoming too much of a 'Jim will fix it' business and that someone else should have a go and so did not go forward again.

One's memories are stirred and all kinds of odd incidents

return. One such matter was a visit of a delegation of Russian fathers who came to consult me on a very serious matter. In Geneva there were several lake-side 'plages', one a very elegant UN place, where the Russians loved to take their children to swim with the rest of the UN families. It seemed that in the USSR, little girls wore swimming shorts without any tops. When the little Soviet lassies saw the other girls wearing bras, they refused to go into the water or undress until they could have bras too. Their mothers were inclined to give in to them, but the fathers thought that if they did they would be departing from their national standards and admitting to a cultural defeat. What advice had I to offer to resolve the problem?

It was wonderful to be consulted on such an important issue by these distinguished bio-medical scientists, a matter involving international relations, peace in the home and the psychological welfare of young people. It was indeed an honour. In a community of men and women from more than ninety nations working together, this kind of thing happened all the time. Small things could blow up into serious issues.

After considerable thought I pronounced judgement. To differ from one's wife on a matter such as this was one thing. One might attempt to enforce male authority, to persuade, to exercise subterfuge or in the last resort to divorce or to simply walk out. But with young women, of say 10 or 11 years of age, particularly since they had formed a collective and had analysed the situation dialectically and had made an iron resolve, in my experience there was only one solution and that was to give in, immediately and gracefully and to admit defeat. I was speaking not only officially but as a father myself of daughters. Being sensible men they agreed.

One of the things that I found in the Staff Training Programme was that the same dichotomy existed between the professional and technical side and the administrative cadre as in the Custom House in Dublin. But here the boot was on the other foot. The WHO was run by doctors, scientists, public health engineers and people like that. More or less the same as exists in most countries in the world which are fortunate enough to remain outside the British system of civil service administration. When the administrative people tried to edge in and grab a little power as they usually do, they were politely slapped down. However, the system was growing a bit long in the tooth and was becoming increasingly difficult to administer, particularly as it had grown so big. There were problems coming up everywhere, which I knew all about as the President of the Staff Association. For example, the staff turnover was too high and it cost far too much to recruit people and place them on station in the field. It was clear that the administrative people could do with some training before the necessary advances on their side of the house could become possible. In any case they were becoming frustrated, since they were a competent lot, very experienced and the financial part of their work was first-class. So, remembering my own experience in the Custom House, and indeed in the interest of the organisation, I suggested that they too should sit around the table by right of their own expertise and not merely be in the background as 'the housekeepers'.

Accordingly I ran a management course for them, brought top-level management people from all over the world to teach them. In a little while, the office walls were covered with PERT diagrams, flow-charts and all kinds of esoteric management curlicues. Now projects on the scientific side were assisted by administrative officers doing operations research studies, cost-benefit analyses, planned programme budgetting, mathematical model-making and other techniques. The scientific people picked up a lot of the techniques and the fact that the administrative side and the scientific side spoke the same language enhanced the work.

This was my life from 1962 to 1967, when my contract ended. Dr Candau asked me to stay on, but I had already had my term prolonged for a year over the official retirement age and I wanted to go home. There were always around WHO a number of 'elder statesmen', old men, who for one reason or other would not give up and go home. They existed on all kinds of small consultancies, some of them more or less working for nothing. It was perhaps because they had no homes to go to being refugees and WHO was their home. I did not want to join their number and so packed up and came home to Dublin.

When I left, Professor Bill Hobson took over as chief of training and with energy and imagination pushed the enterprise on further until he too retired. Then Dr W.L. Barton became Chief. It had been renamed 'The Staff Development and Training Programme' because that in fact was what we had made it. Dr Barton reviewed the work he had accomplished for the period from 1975 to 1982, and showed that in that time he had held 218 training programmes of all kinds, all over the world, which programmes had included 6,933 participants, a magnificent achievement. The baby born in 1962, had by 1982, grown to full maturity.

13

Consultancies

COMING home was something of an anti-climax. I hoped to find a place in a public health department of a medical school, but they were all fully staffed and there was no room for me. I was appointed Lecturer in International Health by UCD but was never asked to give a lecture. Anyway, they all seemed to think that I was too old. I met kindness and friendship everywhere but no one was about to move over in the bed and let me in. Mr Fasenfeld of Antigen Ltd offered me the job of scientific adviser to his company at a handsome salary, but I turned it down as inappropriate.

However, I was appointed Director of the Ambulance Corps of the Order of Malta. This seemed promising and even exciting, as they, the people in the various units, were a wonderful lot. I only held it for a couple of months because I was recalled to Geneva to reorganise the recruiting programme of WHO.

In the recruiting of staff, WHO had a roll of applicants for employment from all over the world. Those whose qualifications and experience might be of use to the organisation were placed on the files. By 1967 these files listed 30,000 candidates and it became increasingly difficult to deal with them. So at the end of 1967, before I had time to settle down at home they brought me back as consultant to help them sort out the problem. I worked out a scheme which enabled us, using the criteria I established, to put the lot on the WHO computer. We took all the material on the 30,000 files relating to applicants and put this data on computer cards or whatever, so that it was in the computer's memory. Then a profile was made out by the unit of the man or woman they wanted, this was fed into the computer, which threw out the files of the people nearest to or matching the profile. From this number a selection was made. Until they had exhausted this selected group, as regards their suitability, the units were not free to do any hiring of other persons.

Early in 1968, I was back again in Geneva, this time to do a 'catalogue of skills' of the staff of WHO. This assignment was an attempt to define what skills were available from the WHO staff. It was of particular importance from the point of future developments. What skills could be said to be 'live'? Which were growing obsolete? Where did we need to supplement skills in areas where we might have future shortages? Later that year, they brought me back to undertake the job of sorting out the 'Consultants List'. These were senior people at the world level, who were recognised as consultants to the World Health Organisation and who would come and advise us, or governments, as world experts. It included people from the Nobel Prize level down to or up to the world's greatest waste disposal expert. There were upwards of 2,000 names on the list and it read like a Roll of Honour of world bio-medical science. The unfortunate thing was that the majority, like myself, were old men or women, whose knowledge was beginning to date a bit. By the time I had finished with them, I had brought the number down to 200. Sadly I had to throw myself out as well. But this started WHO in acquiring a new stock of up-to-date live younger people, old enough to be trusted out to do a job and sufficiently experienced and knowledgeable to be accepted by governments as possessing top-level expertise.

Missionaries

I have always had a thing about Missionaries. I have seen them at work among people of different religions all over the world and have admired them. I had always been interested ever since that wonderful woman, Mother Mary Martin, came to see me in Lurgan, the day after she opened her first Novitiate in Collon, Co. Louth. She asked for my help and we struck up a friendship which lasted till she died.

I tried to stop her building so many hospitals (for about thirty years, she opened a new hospital every year) and urged that in the field, especially in leprosy, she would be better off running a network of clinics to be staffed by native workers, trained by her sister-doctors and sister-nurses. Later she did do this in Nigeria and her leprosy services there were, and are, world models. I brought her sisters to Geneva to meet the world health people and they fell in love with them. Thereafter her services for leprosy were closely linked with WHO.

One day in 1968 when in Armagh visiting my sister Sheelagh, I rang Cardinal Conway and went to see him. I had known him when he was a young professor in Maynooth. I wanted to complain to him about the conditions under which so many Irish missionaries laboured in the field. In Indonesia, I had seen two Irish nuns amongst the Dutch Ursulines, who had not been home for nearly sixty years. I visited Sister Ursuline Savage, a heroine of the Communist revolt in Malang and her sole link with home was her sister, a senior nurse in the Rotunda Hospital. I met a little nun in a French Order in Colombo, who had come from Carlow and who was looking after 150 children with bone and joint TB more or less without trained help. She rarely heard from anyone in Ireland. I told him they had no pensions and if their order could not take care of them they were more or less destitute. Nor was there provision for their care, should their health break down. Years before, I had found out that young men and women were sent out to the tropics without protecting 'shots' and that many had died. While in the Custom House, I had offered help and had been in touch with the Superiors on this. I came away with a request to do a study for him and to write a report on the matter.

The Mission scene in Ireland was most interesting. We had, so far as I could find out at the time, something like 7,000 men and women, Catholic missionaries, all over the world. Most of them were in the Third World. This number did not include Protestant missionaries who were active in the Trinity College Mission of the Church of Ireland and the Presbyterian Qua Ibo Mission and others. The mission effort of Ireland was about the same in size relative to its population, as the American armed forces in Vietnam, when the war was at its peak. Apart from spreading the gospel and preaching peace, they engaged in education, health and development work and their influence on the growth of the Third World was immense.

These people were sent out by more than one hundred different missionary agencies. Each agency recruited, trained or educated personnel, transported them to the mission fields, maintained them, equipped and supplied them. Agencies ranged from the great new missionary orders, through the older orders like the Jesuits, Franciscans and Dominicans down to single small convents running their own little shows in Africa. There were a few lay efforts. None of these agencies seemed to speak to one another and most ran missionary magazines. They were in competition for funds.

A newly consecrated missionary bishop would come home to Ireland and wander around and through his personal contacts would pick up a couple of priests here and a couple of nun-teachers there and a couple of nurses somewhere else and would go back to his new diocese with his catch and in this way would lay the foundation of a Christian community in Africa. Twenty years later there would be a flourishing foundation, a tribute to their heroism and dedication.

When I had done a certain amount of work on the study, I wrote a report for Cardinal Conway and made recommendations. I made a very simple plan to pull the whole thing together, based on the structure of WHO. Each missionary society or agency would join a common organisation, while at the same time preserving its own traditions and autonomy. There would be no compulsion. The organisation would establish a secretariat and a governing council of member organisations, with a rotating membership and which would act as a governing body. The secretariat would provide a base for the training of missionaries in fields of specialist activities and for renewal courses. It would lay down guidelines for health and social care and would consider pension schemes for missionaries and a host of other things. The main objectives being for missionaries to meet, renew, discuss and learn.

The Cardinal looked at the scheme, but did not think that it would work. He said that most of these missionaries belonged to religious orders, which were not subject to control by the bishops. I suggested that if he set the thing up and put in a couple of bishops as presidents or patrons or whatever and then maybe a small 'belt of the crozier' might help to get it going. He went ahead with it and thus the Irish Missionary Union was established.

The Fourth Report on the State of the World Health 1965-1968
Early in 1969, I was asked to come to Geneva to write the
Fourth Report on the World Health Situation covering the
years 1965-8. Each year all the 160 members of WHO send to
Geneva information on the state of the health of the people
in their respective countries. This adds up to an enormous mass
of information. It was collected, categorised and filed by Miss
Pia Monique Elmiger, a Swiss Doctor of Laws from the Sor-
bonne, who did what only the Swiss can do in tabulating,
arranging and sorting out all this stuff.

This information provides the material for a gigantic feed-
back on how the world is going in so far as health is concerned.
Every four years WHO asks someone to sit down, analyse and
make sense out of what has happened during the period. The
first such analysis was carried out by Sir James MacIntosh, a
Scotsman of genius, who had founded the London School of
Hygiene and Tropical Medicine, was its first Director and
played a great part in making it the world-famous institution
it is. The Second and Third were written by Sir John Charles,
former Chief Medical Officer of the Ministry of Health in
London. John Charles had a literary flair and wrote beautifully.
He took great interest in this work and it was a matter of
pride to him to produce something of excellence.

In the analysis of such a vast amount of material, the quality
of the analysis depends on the quality of the data and it is
necessary to check everything. The most interesting aspect
was the search for new patterns of disease, the impact of scientific discoveries and of the new social and economic factors
incluencing health patterns and which might be seen to be
emerging.

I could see a clear picture of improvement; the state of
health of the world was better than before because of the
efforts of the many thousands of people working in the health
fields, for example the world count of two and a half million
nurses. Whether improved social and economic conditions
were of importance or not, the labours of health personnel
were certainly significant. More people were living longer and
enjoying better health than ever before. The changes were
not great but they were to be seen. As regards the great slow
movements and the factors affecting health, the one outstand-

ing factor was the increase in the world's population.

The major developments in the patterns of disease stood out. One was that the parasitic diseases affecting humans had been regarded separately so there were separate campaigns against malaria, or intestinal parasites like hookworm or conditions like bilharzia (the fastest spreading disease at that time, keeping pace with the great irrigation schemes) or indeed of many other diseases. Looking at the overall picture, one could see that there were so many features common to the spread of these diseases that it made more sense to adopt a holistic approach and to seek common denominators in interrupting the spread of transmission

The second was more straightforward. All over the Third World in 1969 a proportion of children were presenting a picture of malnutrition, especially of protein deprivation, with an associated worm infestation, frequent diaorrhoea and often malaria. These things were inter-related and resulted in a lessened immunity, so that a simple upper respiratory infection (for instance the virus of the common cold) could be fatal. Negative nitrogen balance resulted in stunted growth and smaller stature, an inability to learn, and failure to progress at school. It helped to continue the cycle of poverty, of deprivation and of dwelling in slums. The 'syntropy' was linked with the section of the population continuing to live below a reasonable standard of life and included the helpless, the hopeless and those unable to cope. It showed that for future human improvement one must start with the children. This would be the most rewarding approach in health promotion and disease prevention and without it, world poverty could not be solved. Having done the job, I went my way. I always felt that this particular assignment was my 'Olympic medal'.

In the late sixties, I think, an English paediatrician called D.B. Jelliffe, was working in Uganda for WHO and was impressed with the factors of dehydration and depletion of salts as a 'killer' in infant diaorrhoea. He passed fine rubber tubes through the noses of infants with diaorrhoea, these reached down into the stomach. He connected up 'drips' to the tubes, and fluids and salts passed down into the child, restoring the fluid and salts balance of the body. This procedure was of enormous value in saving babies suffering from tropical diaorrhoeas who in a very short time would become dehydrated through loss of body fluids.

When the dreadful situation associated with the independence movement in Bangladesh occurred, I was Chairman of the Staff Association in Geneva. The Staff Associations of the different UN Agencies in Geneva held collections to relieve the distress in that country. I was so ashamed of the meagre amount that our people had contributed which was unusual. At a meeting when it came to my turn to speak, I said that we were working on a project, without revealing the size of our collection. Now we had in WHO a very clever Jugo-Slav called Dr Cvetanocicj, who was Chief of the unit for Bacterial diseases. He had recently devised a fluid pack with which to combat the dehydration found in cholera. This had worked well and was being manufactured in Geneva. It was a life-saver for advanced cases of cholera.

I asked Professor J.P. Dustin of WHO to work a formula for a plastic pack drip which would include amino-acids as well as the fluid and salt replacement. The formula was to be used for kwashiorkor, the final desperate condition in infants and children with protein and calorie malnutrition. Professor Dustin worked very hard on the idea and came up with an appropriate formula. So we presented specimen packs and were given all the UN money to spend. The Swiss manufacturers in Geneva were delighted with the idea and made it for us at cost. I then got the Supplies Group in WHO to organise free transport by Air India and Swissair to Bangladesh.

But you can't be smart all the time. When we checked to see how the packs were being used, we found to our horror that they had been labelled in French and that they lay unused for weeks because the people there did not read French and did not know how and for what they were to be used. But when we sorted this out they worked well.

A short time ago, when looking at the pictures of the Ethiopian Famine on television, I saw a small child with kwashiorkor and one of our packs, being held by his father, while the needle giving the life-fluid was in his arm. I got quite excited at seeing it.

UNICEF is now supplying 25 million small tin-foil packets costing 10 cents each, from central sources, and has organised the manufacture of 20 million more locally. It is thought that 750 million packs are needed as 500 million children suffer each year from diaorrhoea and as said above 5 million die. Hundreds of people all over the world have worked and contributed to research and development in this field but I believe that it all goes back to Jelliffe.

Syria

Although I had removed my name from the role of Consultants, someone put it back on again. So I was recalled from Ireland for another consultancy. The assignment was to take a team to Syria and to find out why malaria, which had been eradicated there, was starting to come back.

We found that Syria had been divided into malaria control districts under medical chiefs and that they were following Sambasivan's protocol of attack, consolidation and maintenance. After years of work all the districts were in the maintenance phase.

The Syrian malaria people had been very successful in the fight against the disease. However, because they had been so successful, they were beginning to relax a bit. The amount of work necessary to find fewer and fewer cases became less rewarding and as well, there was constant pressure to reduce the size of the operation because of the shortage of money. There was also the problem that as malaria came under control, the cooperation the campaign received from the public grew less. My object was to improve the efficiency of the surveillance units. With reduced staffs and so on, the work had become uneven. It was necessary to revitalise the whole operation so as to be able to undertake a final effective operation to ensure that malaria would never come back. With my team we travelled all over Syria, among the Kurds, chasing Bedouin over the desert to examine the mosquitoes in their tents, down the Euphrates and making studies in the valley of the Orontes. A wonderful experience.

As a North of Ireland man, I know a lot about hate and do not like it. In Syria you could literally smell it. It was everywhere. Passing along a lonely desert road, one might see a Bedouin shepherd, sitting on a donkey with his pack and water bag on another ass, streaming out across the desert for maybe a mile would be his flock. But he would be holding his transistor radio close to his ear, listening to programmes of hate for Israel, spewed out from Cairo, Ammon or Damascus. One afternoon, we saw a tremendous parade of armed Palestinians, taking about two hours to pass. One might not be impressed by their military bearing but one was by their bitter, palpable, fanatic hatred.

Travelling Seminar in the USSR

When I got back to WHO in Geneva, I presented the Report on Syria and showed how they could get their malaria problem under control. Soon afterwards the Director of the Division of Medical Education invited me to act as Director of a travelling Seminar to study post-graduate medical education in the USSR.

This was to last one month. There were eighteen participants from seventeen countries. They were mostly Deans of university medical faculties or senior people from Ministries of Health, who were in charge of medical education. As a consequence of the exercise, I was to write a monograph for WHO on post-graduate medical education in the USSR. We were to start in Moscow, then move to Tashkent in Uzbekistan, a day or so in Samarkand and then to Sukhumi, the capital of the Abhkaziayn Autonomous Republic in the Soviet Socialist Republic of Georgia. We would then return to Moscow for a final exercise.

In the ordinary way, the USSR has 77 medical teaching institutes and 9 medical faculties in Universities. They are all under the Ministry of Health of the USSR or the Ministries of Health of the republics in which they are situated. There are 250,000 students and each year 30,000 doctors, dentists and pharmacists qualify. The Ministry of Higher Education decides on educational and social subjects in the curricula and students are expected to learn one foreign language. The post-graduate side was outside of this organisation and included the Central Institute in Moscow and twelve other Institutes throughout the USSR. To give an idea of the size of the operation, the Central Institute had 65 Chairs, 77 full professors, 115 dozents or association professors and 229 lecturers and 9,000 teaching beds. This year before our Seminar, they had given 10,000 doctors post-graduate training and only catered for senior staff. The Russians were very proud of this and wanted to show it off to the world.

When we were all assembled at the Central Institute in Moscow, we were told that we would be addressed by the Director of the International Division of the Ministry of Health and now the Vice Minister to the USSR. When this person arrived complete with entourage, who was it but Dr Tschepin, one of the first group of Russians to arrive in Geneva, one of my pupils and a man I liked very much. When he came first to Geneva he was usually a bit scruffy and had not a tie to his name. Now he was the Chief and Vice-Minister of Health and was treated by everyone with great respect. He welcomed us with an excellent speech in English. I sat back and watched him with pride. He on his side gave WHO credit for his inter-national training and acknowledged the friendship and co-operation that the Russian personnel had received during their service with our Organisation. As well, he made a few flattering remarks about me, which went down well with the group.

During the first few days they gave us a run-down on the health services of the USSR and we visited a lot of institutions in Moscow before leaving for Tashkent.

Here we saw the post-graduate scheme working at a level one step down from Moscow. They had in the main two courses. People first do a correspondence course, very thorough indeed, study the text-books and the literature on the subject, and then write papers, which they submit to the Institute. The second part consists of short residential courses at the Insti-tute. There are full-time courses for specialists, intermittent courses and individual courses. The entire operation was well-run, systematic and there was a wide coverage. As a basic part of a health service and as a means of constantly improving the standard of medicine there was nothing as good as this any-where. Actually it was like a medical Open University except that it was started long before the British version and was on a giant scale.

Everywhere we went in the USSR we came across 'Boss' men. Sometimes it was the Chairman of the committee of the col-lective farm, or the factory manager, or the dean of the medical faculties or whatever. No matter where you go in the world you meet them and there is a great similarity between them. A Chairman of a large collective farm is exactly like an Irish Dáil deputy from a rural constituency. Tough, energetic, sensible, solid men who look after the voters as well as themselves.

So far as we were concerned, the 'Boss' in Abkhazia was the Minister of Health. He took us under his wing and was set to put on a good show. He sailed us up and down the coast in the new national toy, a large hydrofoil, dined us and wined us in the best style and there was never a dull moment. This entertainment was in between our studies and was calculated to assist us in our deliberations.

We flew back to Moscow, where we had more visits. One was of particular interest. It was the Third Medical Institute of Moscow. This did not train doctors, but a broad form of bio-medical scientists. That is in bio-chemistry, bio-physics, electronics, computer sciences, bio-medical engineering and a large range of subjects relating science to bio-medicine. This was new, and we found it interesting and important.

The group then settled down to discuss what we had seen and I was supposed to make notes on this, which I did, and which was to be incorporated into my report and into the monograph which I was to prepare. Most of the people present could have written the report, but when they all gave their views and they argued and discussed them, without any clear purpose, the thing became chaotic, so they left it to me.

A last memory of our Japanese colleague in the group, a senior official of the Ministry of Health, who rarely spoke but who photographed everything all day, every day. When visiting the Third Medical Institute in Moscow, we were shown a Japanese-made scintillometer and were being given an interesting talk on its use by its enthusiastic operator. He rummaged in his capacious camera bag, quietly pushed his way forward and handed the gentleman in charge a catalogue of the new model.

We got back to Geneva, where I wrote up the Seminar, which was published as a Public Health Monograph by WHO. My Russian Co-Director contributed to it by going over the text to examine it for ideological error, a Marxist-Leninist censor theologicus, and he made me change some of it.

14

Two Irish Studies

THERE was still no room for me in the public health academic world in Dublin and as I had had enough running around, I decided to settle down. Tom Barrington, Director of the Institute of Public Administration gave me a desk and facilities in the Institute. After some thought, I decided to do a study of the labour force in Ireland.

Ever since the days of Larcom and Wilde and their distinguished successors down to Lyons, Geary, Donal MacCarthy, Honohan and Linehan, national statistics have been collected with very great accuracy, beautifully presented and then put away and forgotten. Irish statisticians have played a great part in the international development of such parts of this interesting science as national accounts and accounting systems.

In Ireland we had more than ninety trade unions, but while each union was very conscious of its membership numbers and of its own affairs, they did not seem too concerned at that time with the overall labour force or indeed with many aspects of the national social situation. For example, every census for several decades before 1970, had shown that each year, there were 20,000 boys and girls, lost children, who one year after leaving school had still not found a job. This was long before the recent phenomenal rise in unemployment. Following this up, I found that neither the unions or the education authorities at different levels seemed to be aware of this, nor was anything being done for them in any positive way, for example by special apprenticeship or training schemes. Industrialisation was beginning to take root in Ireland, the social structure was changing and it seemed a good idea to try to define 'the Irish Worker' and to secure information from the existing, abundant and excellent material, which had never been examined, and to carry out a demographic study. I analysed the figures from the census returns and many other sources. These were studied by age, sex, occupation, marital status, educational status, geographical distribution and other factors. In fact, a 'model' of the Labour Force. Unemployment and sickness experience in the work force was also examined. A special study was made of man-power in the agricultural sector.

My study showed that the labour force is a dynamic, changing entity, that there is an entry into the labour force and each year a group of people leave it. Clearly the efficiency and morale of this entity is essential to the future welfare of the state.

The study also revealed serious social problems. These were:

1) The existence in 1970 of depressed groups of skilled and unskilled labourers in the lower income groups, with lower levels of education, less security in jobs, seasonal employment, higher unemployment rates amongst people in the groups, higher sickness rates and higher death rates.

2) The existence of a static unemployment situation in 1970 with three-quarters of the unemployed as long-term unemployed and an increasing number of chronic sick people, mainly elderly. Chronic long-term unemployment and chronic sickness were inter-related and mainly affecting the unskilled labouring classes.

3) The existence of a large group of dependants of these two groups. These people had lower standards of living, lesser opportunities and were condemned to perpetuate and suffer poverty as a way of life.

4) A tendency to depend on state assistance; it could be seen that one person in five in 1970 of the total population was maintained wholly or in part by a direct weekly payment by the state.

5) The problem of entry into employment. This had particular reference to school-leavers, drop-outs and the continuing drift of young people into unskilled labouring work.

6) The problem of the elderly, where such a large proportion of those over 60 years are either disabled, unem-

ployed or ineffective as workers and too often prematurely 'worn out' as persons.

7) The large numbers of elderly people suffering prematurely from chronic degenerative diseases, often the final effects of influences which have operated over the preceding years of middle life, either due to work conditions or due to the inability of the health services to deal with them.

8) The changes taking place in occupational groups. For example the sudden disappearance (noticeable already in the 1970s) of 5,000 grocer's 'curates' in a few years, due to the advent of the supermarkets. This group was sunk without either trace or comment.

I have listed eight problems, but the main finding was that we had a live, active, healthy labour force, as a positive entity, that it needed care, that it represented a large number of human beings, that it was dynamic and changing, that it was continually becoming better educated and that it was a potent force for the future development of the state and our nation.

The study was published as a book in 1971 by the Institute of Public Administration under the title of *The Irish Worker*. I was disappointed with the book's lack of impact. It did not really do anything for the group of poor and underprivileged, unskilled people, the chronic sick, the chronic unemployed, who, in the end, were the people I was really trying to help. Possibly it was a bit before its time, possibly too academic or whatever but it did define the problem and possibly started people thinking. But it did not 'sell' the concept of a labour force as an entity, as something to be cherished as a vital part of society, as something to be educated, tuned to an optimum pitch of efficiency and responsibility and concerned for the nation's welfare. It did have an effect however in that the Central Statistics Office now publishes an annual survey of the labour force.

A Year in Fanad

When I was finished my study of the labour force, I was at a loose end and restless. I could have organised more work in Geneva and gone back to WHO, but I had had enough of travel-

ling. Equally, I did not want to start up our farm in Portmarnock again. The city was moving out on top of us and it was
not going to be as pleasant to live there in future as when it
had been a quiet rural community.

In August 1970, I was driving to Sessiagh in Donegal, where
my brother Donnell had a fishing lodge on the Lough, hoping
to have a few days fishing, when going through Lifford, I had
a brain wave. A few days before, I had seen an advertisement
for a dispensary doctor for Fanad, the long peninsula stretch-
ing north between Lough Swilly and Mulroy Bay. I turned the
car off the road, went to the County Hall and asked had they
recruited anyone yet for Fanad. It seemed that no one wanted
to work in such a remote place as Fanad. They had to get
someone, since Dr MacMenamin, the incumbent, was 78 and
his family insisted that he should retire. A couple of weeks
later, after a selection board, I was appointed. I went up,
found a holiday chalet to rent in Portsalon, moved in and
started to work.

I wanted to do a study of a rural community, to describe
its structure and how it worked. A further aim was to present
and define its problems as a community, its resources, how
they were being used, to work out socio-economic indicators
and the possible role of the community in planning and
development. In short, part input-output analysis and part
situational analysis. The fact that it was part Gaeltacht was
an added bonus.

Dr MacMenamin was a remarkably spry old man. He had
been there for more than fifty years and was universally
beloved, in fact he was an example of the best that Ireland
could offer in the way of a country doctor who cared for the
people. We made an arrangement that he would continue to
look after private patients, which gave him something to do,
while I occupied myself with the dispensary patients. This
gave me enough to live on and time to do my study. The dispensary was moved out of Dr MacMenamin's house and across
the road to two rooms behind the post office in Tamney village. I ordered equipment and medicines through the county
council and on 1 October 1971 I was in business.

In an ordinary rural area, the medical expectation of the
dispensary population, i.e. those entitled to free medical care,

was not high. There were two dispensary days a week, when
the dispensary was open for an hour or two in the morning, with
the district nurses in attendance. Patients could get national
health insurance certificates to say that they were incapable
of work through illness, new cases were seen, chronic patients
received 'repeats' of their medicines. As part of the tradition of
Irish rural medicine, there was of course also extensive home
visiting of patients and a close relationship with people. There
was a particularly easy-going association between Dr Mac-
Menamin and his patients, who came whenever they wanted
or sent for him at any hour they liked, 24 hours a day, seven
days a week. On the other hand they were so fond of him that
this was not abused, or at least not often.

Although I had Dr MacMenamin to hold my hand should I
meet anything with which I could not cope, I was somewhat
nervous at the beginning, since I had not examined a patient
seriously for nearly thirty years. Dr MacMenamin on the other
hand, after fifty years' experience, could spot a sick man or
woman from 100 yards away and have a diagnosis made before
they could come face-to-face with him.

So to be on the safe side, lest anyone should drop dead on
the way home from the dispensary, I examined every patient
very carefully. This was much to the amusement of the two
district nurses. However I got my own back on them by starting a clinic for ante-natal examination of mothers, for child
care, including weighing babies and so on, and for immunisation of children.

I went along happily with this for a few weeks, when the
word went around Fanad on the very effective grapevine,
that 'this new man really examines you'! Now if you examine
enough people you are bound to find someone with an abnormal condition, which they have put up with, but which can
be cured. So again the word went around that 'the new man
finds things and tries to cure them', so trade increased, until
instead of a couple of hours in the morning, the dispensary
session became a day-long affair. Dr MacMenamin watched
the whole performance with amusement, since the same thing
had happened to him, when he began in Fanad fifty years
before.

Fanad is extraordinarily beautiful, with Lough Swilly, the

Lake of the Shadows, on one side with the light changing from moment to moment and with the views of the great sweep of the Inishowen mountains and the rocky heads of Malin and Dunaff. And on the other side Mulroy Bay with lovely wooded islands. I was home. There was an added attraction in that at the south of the district were the Knockalla Mountains (the Mountains of the Swans) beyond which was the great glen, Glenvar. This was full of Deenys and indeed my grandfather Deeny had built the church there. This and the little port of Rathmullan, was Deeney and Deeny country and I was amongst my own.

What really made it home were the people. One day, I went up Glen Fanad and through winding lanes gradually climbing up the mountainside came to a small mountain farm. The daughter of the house had asked me to come to see her baby. She had been a long-distance bus conductress for years on the run between Glasgow and Edinburgh and had married and come home with her man. When I had examined the child, she explained that she wanted her father down off the hill so that I could take his blood-pressure. I watched him come down, leaping like a young goat.

I looked at the view and could see the wonderful coast line of north Donegal and unusually, the Stacks on Tory Island and the Horns on Horn Head. It was breath-taking. Looking around, the small farm was neat and tidy, the farm-yard clean, the house well-thatched and there was an old but well-cared-for tractor. When her father finally arrived he was not out of breath or fussed and greeted me as one gentleman to another and asked me would I sign his 'Old IRA' pension form. I said I would if he would let me take his blood-pressure, which I knew he did not want. He agreed. He was well over seventy years of age and his blood pressure was normal. He was as hard and as tough as a piece of old oak with a leather cover. We then had an easy chat. After a short word on the great qualities of the Deenys, which pleased me very much, and further considerations on life in general and the iniquities of the government and a touch on religion, I started for the door. Before I left I turned and asked, 'do you drink much whiskey?'. He replied, 'only when I go to the cattle mart at Milford, then I might have seven or eight, I always drink Scotch, but mind you I always come home in a taxi'.

Going down that mountain, I realised that what I had seen was a completely free man, something unique in Europe. He was master of his own piece of land, owed no one anything, could take a day off when he felt like it, without asking anyone's permission or seeking a sick certificate. He had fought for his country's freedom, believed in God and without worrying too much about it, was quite satisfied that he was on the right road to Heaven. He stood firm and free and was economically, socially and spiritually secure. In Fanad, many people were like that and I loved them.

The people of Fanad were descendants of the gallowglasses; these were men from the south west of Scotland and from the Isles who came to fight for O'Neill and O'Donnell in their wars against the English. Later as they came over in greater numbers they filtered down through the country and became an important part of the standing armies of the Gaelic Chieftains.

One evening in Fanad, when doing a sick-call nearby, I went down to an old MacSweeney ruined tower at a pool, 'Between the Waters', and got out of the car and sat down on a stone to enjoy the sunset. Suddenly I heard a noise, a creak of oars and a galley made its way in quietly and people landed, big men and their women and children, laughing and shouting in Gaelic. It was a mystic experience; a dream, a Campbell, Clann ua Duibhne galley of galloglaich coming in. I shook it off and got up and went home. Such things are dangerous for Irishmen — it leads them to their deaths from hunger strikes, forlorn hopes or rebellion.

In Fanad more than half of the people bore one of twelve family names, Carrs or Kerrs, Friels, Sweeneys, MacAteer or MacEntyre, and Coyles or Colls. There was a pervasive family network and everyone was related by blood or marriage to everybody else. Over the years they had established Fanad colonies in Glasgow, Liverpool, Corby, Bristol, Philadelphia, Boston and Dublin. There they were solid citizens, obsessed with education as were those who remained at home. They became policemen, teachers, contractors in earthmoving work, steel erectors, tunnellers, builders, priests and nuns. In Fanad they were excellent stockmen and reared good cattle on the hills. On the small amount of fertile ground they specialised in the raising of seed potatoes.

Fanad was a community of hard-working small farmers with a total population of 2,700 souls. The community was burdened with a high dependency rate of children and old people. The social services, such as rural electricity, piped water supplies, owner occupied houses, roads and so on were very good indeed for such a remote part of Europe. Support services, such as dole for small farmers with non-viable holdings, old age and sickness pensions and other provisions for the needy, were fully effective. There were two district nurses and the family network ensured that old people were well cared for. The education services both primary and secondary were first class. There was no crime, no alcoholism, and a serene way of life. While they were happy and enjoyed their lives enormously, they were at the same time abstemious to the point of austerity and maintained the old gaelic tradition of the hearth swept bare and tidy. They were great savers and great survivors. They must not be thought of as a backward isolated group, since they travelled incesssantly, visiting relatives in the Fanad communities abroad, going to football matches, political meetings and so on. When I checked with the Post Office I found that they sent and received more than a quarter of a million letters during the year 1970.

Over the generations they had saved, and one way or another possessed quite a bit of money. For example, there was more than £1.5 million on deposit in a bank in the neighbouring town. This was in one bank. There it was saved, perhaps from people returning from the US or the life savings of some small mountain farmer, or the hoard, which some old bachelor policeman had accumulated during his life-time of service. Through the operation of the banking system, £1.5 million on deposit generates five times this amount in credit for investment. The tragedy was that this money was being used for investment and development by the banks, for any place except Fanad. Meanwhile Fanad stagnated.

Because of the high dependency rate in the community, the various social services cost the government (both central and local) about £250,000 pounds a year for the area. The people earned almost £300,000 from agriculture, nearly £200,000 from tourism and from money sent from outside of Fanad and from home crafts such as knitting. It cost a little over £500,000 for them to live, pay for agricultural inputs, house-building and such things. The balance, £150,000 they saved.

Formerly they produced stone (for instance granite square setts for the Liverpool streets), chemicals such as iodine from seaweed, linen and other things, but these industries had perished. So this clever hard-working sturdy community stagnated, with a constant drain of young, well-educated people leaving because of lack of opportunity. Meanwhile the banks held enough of their money to transform the place.

During the year I got together a local group, headed by Sean Dorrian a school teacher and we set up a Fanad Development Association. We planned first to build a Community centre which would, we hoped, form the focus for a Gaelic Summer School. A football ground and sports amenity was laid out and things began to happen. People who had never had a chance before, showed what they could do. Years later, I went back and found that they had built one of the finest community centres in Ireland, had a Festival of Fanad going and the whole morale of the place, so far as this kind of thing counted, had changed. Indeed with Father Sweeney as coach, their football team achieved a national final.

The pleasure of fishing for sea-trout on Sundays with a good friend Mr Griffith, a carpenter in the neighbouring Milford Bakery, woke me up to the possibility of using Mulroy Bay for fish farming. I visited Bord Iascaigh Mhara in Dublin and asked them to investigate the matter. Then we all got tangled up together. The local fishermen wanted an ice-plant and something done for their neglected harbour. BIM and the County Development Authority wanted a crab fishing and crab-meat packing project. I wanted a cooperative for the Fanad-Rosguil fishermen and to start a scallop and oyster development project in Mulroy Bay. This was to be only a start and for me it was important that they should get control of their own waters and should have a winter fishing ground in shelter and not to have to drown themselves in the Atlantic storms in small boats using rotten little rocky inlets, so-called harbours, with half the time, wind and tide making them inaccessible. Years later, after I left, they sorted it all out and there is now a first-class shell-fish and particularly salmon enterprise in Mulroy Bay.

Dr MacMenamin and I did a small study of the case-load of work for a month to try to discover the type and amount of sickness in the community. We performed 716 services between us during the month; 341 were home visits and there were 375 attendances either at his house or at the dispensary. We found that there was a very large number of chronic chest conditions, not tuberculosis, but a surprising number for such an otherwise healthy community. They were probably some unusual form of 'Farmer's Lung', possibly from mouldy hay.

After a year in Fanad my study of the area was complete. I had made a socio-economic 'profile' of the community and one of the best years of my life was over. I had learnt enough Irish to carry on a simple conversation, had bought a cottage and was prepared to settle there for life. However, it was too remote for my family. As they were all against it, I resigned my post and came South again.

Studies like this have been one of the interests of my life. I have always had a pot quietly simmering away on the side while I got on with the ordinary bread and butter tasks for which I was being paid. These were a series of investigations which I carried out myself or with help from others. They began about 1936 and have continued for fifty years and in fact I have just completed a little job for WHO on 'Conflict in Health Systems'.

Without any planning or anything else, there was a kind of sequence in these studies. Counting them in a rough way, there seems to have been nearly one for every year. The first were the local ones done in Lurgan, and then the infant mortality study in Belfast was a bit bigger and more ambitious. When I moved to Dublin, they became national; later in Geneva they were either national or international and finally, the report on the world health situation was global.

In the great majority of these studies, what I had actually done in each case was to make a medico-social 'model'. Now, when I started I had never heard of models nor at that time, starting more than fifty years ago, had anyone else. The idea of models and modelling was to come later. The concept nowadays embraces all techniques which lead to a simplified more explicit description of a real situation.

Sir Karl Popper, to my mind the greatest living philosopher, has been interested in this field and in an analysis of the aims of science deals with models. He says that the main aim of science is to find satisfactory explanations of whatever strikes us as being in need of explanation. Explanations in the social sciences are very similar to certain physical explanations, but problems of explanation in the social sciences give rise to problems not encountered in the physical sciences. Since social sciences must be studied under typical conditions and situations, the construction of models is the best approach. He emphasised that social scientists should construct models by 'Situational Analysis', which provides models (perhaps rough and ready) of typical social situations. Popper stated in 1967, when he published the concept, that this is the only way to explain what happens in society. I entitled my study in Fanad, which was an input-output examination model, published in 1973, 'A Situational Analysis'.

My good fortune was that I hit upon this model-making idea in 1938 and developed it in all kinds of ways in the medical-social field. Looking back on it, I did not really know what I was doing. It was only over the years that in the field of science people came to appreciate what models were all about.

I found that it was a technique which could be used by a general practitioner, without resources, working in a small town. In fact it was because I had no laboratory, university or government backing, that I had to work out this kind of thing for myself.

Later on, I found that it could be used to solve problems in my work in the Irish civil service. In my hands, certainly in the beginning, it was simple and possibly a bit homespun, but it worked. All you needed, when you had decided what you wanted to do, was a kind statistician who would advise you on the material you were going to collect, so that it was capable of analysis.

Some time later, Telefis Eireann became interested in the economic situation in Fanad as shown by my study, which had been published in *Administration* in 1973. We made a documentary on the community. This enabled me to confront the bankers publicly and to demand that they should give something back to the people whose money they held and used to their own profit. I wanted them to start some form of development project, operated for the benefit of the Fanad people and managed on their behalf by the bank or banks, but nothing happened. However the Development Association of the Fanad people themselves is doing good work particularly in tourism and of course the Mulroy mariculture has been a success.

15

The Vatican 1971-72

I HAD now three houses: one in Portmarnock, a farm in Wexford and a cottage in Donegal. I put the farm in Wexford up for sale, but got no offers and so decided to sell our place in Portmarnock where we had lived for thirty years. I had had enough of Dublin and enjoyed the life in Donegal, so could not go back to urban life. Another powerful factor influencing these decisions was the view of the bank manager, who had started to act up a bit.

So I sold Portmarnock with a good deal of sorrow but if I was to enjoy retirement, the farm in Rosslare was the place to be. On the day of the sale, I got a message from the Papal Nuncio, with an invitation to dinner the next evening.

After the excellent dinner which Nuncios always serve, Dr Alibrandi, whom I had known in Indonesia, produced a letter from Cardinal Villot, the Secretary of State in the Vatican. This instructed him to invite me to accept a post as Scientific Advisor to the Holy See, assuring me of his best sentiments and mentioning, by the way, that the salary would not be large. So I told the Nuncio that I would have to think about it.

It was all very inconvenient, but in my book, when the Pope calls you to his service, you go. So I rang the Nuncio the next morning, accepted the post and awaited instructions.

The last couple of years had been interesting. The Ministry of Health of the USSR, the Dublin Institute of Public Administration, WHO, Syria, Fanad, and now the Vatican. I was getting around. As a good Irish general practitioner, I was seeing the spread of my practice.

When I got to Rome, I found out what it was all about. Pope Paul VI had instituted three great councils. These were partly because he felt they were needed, and partly to implement the findings of Vatican II. One was the Council of the Laity, which was to be the instrument to develop the participation of the laity in the organisation and life of the Catholic Church. The second was the Council for Justice and Peace. This was the instrument which would harness the interest and activities of the hundreds of millions of Catholic people all over the world in pursuit of justice whether social or political, and of peace. The third which had just been established, was Cor Unum, (One Heart), the Pontifical Council for Human and Christian Development. I was concerned with this one.

Briefly, the Holy Father had become worried about Catholic charities. Some had become positively embarrassing to him. They had achieved notoriety in the Biafran War, where some religious had zealously espoused the cause of the Ibo people with an enthusiasm which might have prejudiced the position of Catholics elsewhere in Nigeria. In the Sudan, they were believed to be concerned in the Anyanya rebellion. Many of the great charities were a law unto themselves, but it was important that the Church should know what they were doing, and that somehow their activities should be coordinated. Another factor was the many different ways in which new African states, for example, were receiving aid or not receiving it. This was having all kinds of odd effects, political, social and cultural. It was desirable that Catholic charitable support should be part of an overall national development, related to the Catholic Church in the country but integrated on an ecumenical basis with other aid efforts.

Three of us were given the job of sorting the thing out. The Secretary of the Council and the head of our group was Father de Riedmatten, a Swiss Dominican, whom I had known in Geneva, where he had been the Representative of the Holy See accredited to the UN. He was something of a diplomatic genius and had three Doctorates, from Freiburg, from Oxford and from Rome. The other colleague was Monsignor Kada, a Hungarian who had been all over the world as a Papal diplomat. He is now an Archbishop. He was charming, intelligent and spoke many languages. In addition he was young and cheerful.

No one ever told me why I was chosen. It seems that for such a post as this, three names are submitted to the Pope. He puts a tick after the name he chooses and writes 'sta bene' and that's that.

As ours was a new enterprise, we were given an office in the Vatican proper on a long galleria or stone corridor with walls lined with inscribed stones from classical times, coming from all over the early civilised world.

The Vatican civil service was like nothing I had seen before. I had, one way or another, witnessed the insides of many governments particularly their health departments, but this place was different. The Curia's thought processes were unique. Time did not seem to matter, and there was a sublime certainty about everything they did. After all, if you have been in business for 2,000 years, a month or so, one way or another doesn't count. Also working for the Lord does seem to create an atmosphere of security and certainty. For outsiders, the Curia has always had a sinister and intolerant reputation. A smell of the Inquisition, of theologians being kicked about, of intrigue, of fiddling bishoprics and benefices, of selling indulgences, excommunications, annulments, of vatican lawyers, investigative journalists finding skullduggery and of Rome rule. Working there and as an experienced observer you soon find that today this is nonsense. The place is quite ordinary in its way.

I never saw a place where they got so much work done and used so little paper. Nothing circulating inside ever went beyond a single sheet and even then the text was usually limited to a few lines. The top part of a memorandum, if it was going up the line, started with salutations and then titles. Eminentissimo, Reverendissimo, Excellentissimo, Illustrissimo and after that their territorial designations, Bishop or Archbishop of this, that or the other. I qualified unofficially for Illustrissimo, a courtesy I appreciated and which amused me, but which I did not deserve. Someone might be Titular Archbishop of X, a former thriving city in Byzantium with a glorious history of religion, art and culture. Maybe when I was in Syria, I had seen it as a 'tel' with a few mud huts on top of the mound, literally a huge 'kitchen midden', but its story kept alive down through the ages by a line of Christian archbishops, now possibly the doyens of the diplomatic corps in some country.

At the bottom of the memorandum, there were more salutations. For someone really important, there could be four full lines at the top. Then it was always typed very carefully on thick paper, never folded, placed in a huge envelope and delivered by hand by our sergeant. They did things in style in the Vatican. Things like stationery, office equipment and supplies were first-class and the whole operation was a model of efficiency and cleanliness. Nevertheless the Vatican was run on a shoe-string.

In another way, the Vatican was unique in its form of administration, being operated by clever men, working hard but thinking in and speaking a different language from say the ordinary international organisation. As an example, the First Synod after Vatican II picked up the fact that there was no statistical organisation available in the Holy See and suggested quietly that it was time that they had one. So, like all Vatican projects it started in a very small way. The staff included Monsignor Norese, a fine scholar and Professor D'Agata, part-time. He was Professor of Statistics in the University of Rome. I was roped in to give a hand.

None of the Curia had any money. Some, like Monsignor Kada were keeping widowed mothers. They were mostly people who belonged to religious orders and lived cheaply in the monasteries belonging to their orders. Even the cardinals resident in Rome were relatively poor men and any surplus cash they had went in all sorts of charitable ways such as paying on the quiet for young seminarians to eke out an existence while they studied in some college. In addition to the work they did in the Vatican, many had other jobs such as teaching in some of the Papal Universities in Rome. A few only had small cheap cars. Once in a while if they got their hands on some money, they promptly 'blew it' on a good dinner. It was a delight to dine with such people. They were excellent hosts, great company and the talk was always good.

While Father de Riedmatten was organising the office and before Monsignor Kada arrived, I started out to get some idea of the lie of the land. I found that world-wide there were more than 1,000 major Catholic charitable organisations including for example nearly 140 national Caritas Societies. I estimated that each year the Catholic charities collected more than £400 million. Some countries collected huge sums, for instance the West German bishops in a single appeal always raised more than £20 million. On the other hand there were no priorities or planning in the spending. There was over-lapping and people applying for aid might apply to a dozen organisations and receive help from several or none, depending on the presentation and the pathos of the appeal.

Of course those in charge of the various agencies were very well aware of all this and were doing something about it. Professor Van Istandael, who occupied a Chair at Louvain University, had set up an organisation to begin to coordinate things and had a computer to process applications. He had as assistant a young Irishman, Brian MacKeown, who now runs Trocaire, the national Catholic overseas aid organisation operated by the Irish Hierarchy.

While some of the heads of these greater charities could be described as prima donnas, in the main they were sensible, highly experienced and very dedicated. They were also scared of the Vatican and what we were up to. It was the same story as the relations between the Department of Health in Dublin, the Irish county councils and the medical profession. The charities had autonomy, were fiercely national, had the money and would spend it more or less as they wished. They did not welcome the Holy Father, much less the Curia, telling them what to do.

But a Provisional Council had been established by the Pope and the first meeting had been called. Our big task was to get ready for it and to organise it in such a way that something worthwhile would come out of it.

As the time drew on, Father de Riedmatten, Monsignor Kada and I went out to a Jesuit monastery in the Alban Hills outside of Rome and spent a week-end planning our strategy. Father de Riedmatten had a splendid schedule laid out and, being Swiss, wanted everything to go with efficiency and promptness, sticking to an exact time-table. This was important as we had very little money and to keep the Council a day extra in Rome would be expensive. Monsignor Kada, the diplomat, in anticipation of the opposition, was concerning himself with creating the right atmosphere of cooperation and friendliness. My experience with the Irish county councils and difficult groups such as the UN Staff Associations led me to suggest that we should begin with a period of catharsis. We should give the members of the Council the floor, when they would do the talking, express their views and get the rancour and opposition out of their systems. Everyone should have an opportunity to speak. Then when they had quietened down, we might hit them with the inadequacy of their various operations and their lack of system and direction. From the technical point of view, my aim was to impress on the Council the need to swing their approach to planned development and programmes with defined goals and targets, in an endeavour to achieve something tangible and lasting.

When the Council assembled, it was seen to be a formidable lot with a plethora of Cardinals, Archbishops, Bishops and so on down to lay experts from all over the world. The first session was opened by Cardinal Villot, the Secretary of State, who set the note by saying that the Holy Father was determined to put order into the whole field of Catholic charity, to coordinate the various interests and to have them work together. Then we threw the ball to the members, and it was a revelation. The Holy Father had acted very wisely in calling them together. For example, it was literally astonishing to find how many programmes had become meshed with their country's official Government aid. Archbishop Gleeson, head of the Australian charities, for instance, made it clear that their work was integrated into Australian government projects in Papua and New Guinea and that this arrangement was satisfactory and, by implication, was not to be disturbed. It was difficult sometimes to see whether governments were exploiting Catholic aid, or that Catholic aid was being used independently or even against governments. Each and everyone spoke and they all had different slants and attitudes. When they all had voiced their opinions and objections, they quietened down and listened to us.

As the Vatican technical expert I presented to them a global analysis of their programmes and it was pointed out that they must coordinate their efforts and set themselves targets in each country in which they were working. They were told that their approach was too fragmented and too broad, that they should determine priorities and stick to them and set objectives and measure their progress towards achieving them and much more. Actually they knew all this, but had never been able to come together and hear an objective and rigorous evaluation of what they were doing, based on their own reports and presented in a reasonable and sympathetic manner.

When they saw that we were not threatening their freedom of action they began to work well. The group included people of very great ability and experience and wisdom and it was a pleasure to hear them. They agreed with and gradually accepted the need for a more positive approach and their collective experience and ideas enhanced anything we put before them. All we did was to provide the setting, the magnificence of a Vatican Council Chamber, give the thing a bit of a push, and they did the work. Our task in the end was relatively minor, as it was meant to be. We ended up with an excellent Report to the Holy Father.

At the end, there was a formal presentation of the Report to the Pope. There is a story about this. A few days before he was to meet them, the Holy Father sent notes to us on an address he proposed to give them and asked us to draft it. There arrived six pages of notes, written in the small beautifully rounded handwriting of the Pope himself. Our office 'scrittore' a lawyer, translated them for me and I was asked to have a go. Impressed by the dignity of the occasion and the person for whom I was acting I did my best. It was tidied up properly and sent in. It came back in a few hours and we were told to try again. This time all three of us worked on it. It went in and came back even quicker. We tried again and again failed. Finally we were told enough is enough. When he did give his address it bore no relation to anything we had tried to produce. If anything it was a distillation of his own original notes. The real point of this story is to give an example of the incredible industry of Pope Paul VI. I've never seen anyone work quite so hard as he did. Yet he was completely human. He cared for the people who worked for him. Little messages of appreciation would come down, you would be told of some remark that he had made about you; apart from seeing him very occasionally and then always in a group, you felt that there was a recognition of your existence.

It was the same thing in the Secretariat. Cardinal Villot and Archbishop Benelli, the Sosstituto, sent for you from time to time, and opened up discussions on your work. These would then broaden out and they would invite views on all kinds of matters. It was much more than mere politeness, there was an understanding and something like appreciation in a decent kind of way. Here was I with my Mother and Child Scheme at one time condemned by the Irish hierarchy as being against Christian teaching, calmly advising the Holy Father on the dispensing of the entire Catholic charity of the world. I was still unrepentantly proclaiming that the lives of children and mothers should be saved and made more healthy and rewarding by public health and organised medicine and indeed by Christian mass action. In an odd kind of way and of course inspired by the Holy Spirit, Mother Church can be very wise, even with so minor a character as myself.

At the request of some of the delegates, after the Council was over I started a series of case-studies. These were to show how Christian aid could be provided for certain developing countries. On the ground, there were excellent relations with other churches, so the approach was ecumenical and was to integrate Christian aid with UN aid, with unilateral aid direct from governments and with the programmes of the governments themselves. These ideas and studies went, some to people like Bishop James Sangu in Tanzania and some to await the consideration of the next Council. I also prepared a Directory of the major Catholic aid organisations, what they did and what were their resources. This had been requested by the first Council as they had no idea of how many agencies existed and where they were located.

In many ways, life was interesting in the Vatican. The Mensa, or senior staff canteen, was the Pope's Table, a sort of mediaeval survival. The food was simple, of good quality and cheap. It was mostly used by Vatican lawyers, artists or journalists on the staff of the Osservatore Romano and the senior scrittores. The Vatican Pharmacy was up to the best international standards and was staffed by Australian Brothers of St John of God, who were all qualified pharmacists. The 'Anon' was a very large supermarket, which supplied all the workers in the Vatican state, the religious houses in Rome and a number of the local poor, who for one reason or another had the privilege of shopping there. It was non-profit, tax-free and cheap. The control over who should shop there was very tight since the Roman business world objected to it.

An incident that sticks in my memory was the Christmas midnight mass, celebrated by the Holy Father in the Sistine Chapel. This was for the 'Family of his Household', and for the diplomats accredited to the Holy See. It was an impressive affair, with the Swiss Guards in their especial finery with red feathers in their helmets, polished steel breastplates and a great shine on their halberds. Then the diplomats parading in, some in fancy uniforms or national dress with the sashes and star or crosses of their orders and decorations, all a-glitter. Their wives followed demurely in black, with mantillas and the odd diamond showing. The Sistine choir singing away and the whole place ablaze with light while the Holy Father said the first of his three Christmas masses and gave Holy Communion to his 'Family'. The second is said at dawn in a traditional church in a poor district of Rome and the third in state in St Peter's at 10 o'clock. A heavy load for an old man.

The experience which touched me most deeply in Rome was in the Vatican. The Holy Father Paul VI decided to consecrate seventeen Bishops and Archbishops in one ceremony in St Peter's. When they were assembled I saw a small Indian wearing a cope in colours usually associated with the Buddhist theme of the spectrum of the rainbow. A tall blond man, to be consecrated as the Bishop in the Ukranian Rite of their Community in Latin America was wearing a great golden byzantine crown. Outstanding because of his height and presence was the late Dermot Ryan to be consecrated as the Archbishop and Metropolitan of Dublin.

In fact it was a great day for the Irish, since Cardinal Conway sat at the Pope's side on the altar. President Hillery occupied an honoured place.

The long consecration ceremony in St Peter's proceeded, when suddenly there was a pause and an ancient cardinal, who must have been 90, got to his feet and tottered down the aisle and proceeded to lay his hands on the heads of those being consecrated. The old man could hardly stand, but made his way bravely from the one to the other, possibly his last defiant act of faith. He was followed by a few others almost as old and then there emerged a small flood seeming to number hundreds, of cardinals, archbishops, bishops and abbots of all races from all over the earth, all slowly and deliberately passing on what they themselves had received. It had gone on, back through the ages, from generation to generation, back to Jesus Christ our Saviour himself. This was truly the Apostolic Succession.

Having seen through the setting up of the Council and of the programme to be followed and having carried out the case-studies and other tasks, I decided that I should go home. Since we had sold the house in Portmarnock and needed to make the move to Rathdowney in Wexford, I took my leave. The Holy Father presented farewell gifts to my wife, a gold and mother of pearl rosary, and to me — a medal of himself and a set of engravings of the Raphael paintings in the Stanza Segnatura and a letter of thanks for my work. So that was that job finished.

16

Rathdowney, Rosslare,
County Wexford 1971

WE SETTLED down in Rathdowney House at Rosslare.
This was a late Georgian house on 125 acres of land and
had been the site of an old mediaeval castle or tower and before
that a Gaelic rath; the place had been inhabited for over 2,000
years. There was a belt of trees around the house and it stood
on the first bit of high ground on the east side of the great
south slobs of Wexford harbour. It was a few miles from the
port of Rosslare, and a mile or so from the lovely Rosslare
beach. Taking everything into consideration, the place was
just right for us.

One of Rathdowney's charms was the fact that this part of
the world had formerly been an important focal point of the
mediaeval Angevin empire, guarding the southern end of the
Irish Sea and providing an entry into Ireland. The mediaeval
atmosphere still lingered and the old farm buildings might
have been in Normandy. However, the old farm buildings
soon lost their charm. After I had spent three weeks with a
fork, clearing manure out of the cattle sheds, I soon found
that the day of 'mixed farming' had gone and that to survive
one had to have a specialty.

So I became a hard-working practical farmer, put up some
modern buildings and a silage installation and went into grass-
fed cattle. We wintered and fattened 100 head of cattle each
year. I found a new pleasure in doing things like laying concrete, driving the tractor, in practical grass growing operations
and the winter feeding of the cattle. At the same time, the
garden became a great interest. The serenity, tranquility and
so on was wonderful. The hard work, fresh air and exercise
was extremely healthy and the constant anxiety of trying
to make a living and to keep from going broke kept you on
your toes. To make a complete change in one's way of life,

to develop a range of new interests and to make new friends gave us fifteen years of happiness and an added dimension to our lives which I never expected to achieve.

Ombudsman in Geneva

Apart from the odd short trip for such things as working parties in Rome or such places, I was determined to stay where I was and to enjoy Rosslare. However another call came. One night Dr Mahler, the Director-General of WHO rang me and asked would I come to Geneva and act as Ombudsman for WHO.

What had happened was this. WHO Headquarters staff had for some unknown reason become increasingly on edge, there was frustration, a malaise, an accidie, a lowering of morale which showed itself in a vague general unhappiness. Many felt that they should have an Ombudsman. Mahler asked me to do the job, since it seemed that the staff had remembered the fatherly care I took of them years before as Chairman of the Staff Association.

The staff were delighted to have an Ombudsman produced for them, but the administrators were somewhat ambivalent, since my appointment more or less implied criticism of them. So firstly I had to convince the administration that I was not a threat to them. Secondly that I should try to settle as many cases as possible myself and reserve the big stick of the Director-General's intervention for situations which could not be resolved in any other way. Thirdly and most important of all, that I should seek to find an added dimension in each case of trouble which would enable me to break the deadlock, see fair play and settle the matter amicably.

Part of the malaise stemmed from the peculiar position of these international civil servants. Because they were expatriate, without roots or real participation in the local Genevois society, because they had high standards of living, were constantly mobile and because they were introverted, being only concerned with themselves, their tasks and their organisation, and for many other reasons, the members of the WHO community were subject to stresses and strains which they themselves did not appreciate. In fact the assignment turned out to be far more a counselling responsibility than that of a straight-forward Ombudsman checking files for administrative injustices. While the appointment was itself a benefit, after a year's hard work, so many problems were solved that there was not the need for a full-time Ombudsman. I became part-time, working alternate months. Later it was possible to hand it over to a capable successor, John Burton.

One winter evening, coming over the Jura mountains, as I descended the pass, I stopped to enjoy the view. Here and there in the mountains were the small clusters of lights of the mountain villages, some in France and some in Switzerland. They represented mountain communities, little changed since the middle ages and enjoying a tranquil, rural way of life. Down in the valleys were small industrial towns. Their lights showed small factories and shops representing another kind of community, the industrial. Their small economies, their products and employment determine the life-style of the inhabitants.

Looking towards Geneva, one could see the buildings of the agencies of the United Nations ablaze with lights, like great ocean liners; the World Health Organisation, the International Labour Office, the World Telecommunications, the World Meteorological and others, and finally the great constellation of lights from the Palais des Nations. These were the post-industrial communities and this was a kind of lesson of Time. This view and the thoughts that it inspired, produced some ideas. While I was on this job I did a sociological study of the Geneva Headquarters staff of WHO and prepared a paper which I read to the WHO University of Geneva Medical Society.

Rome

My last job involving travel was unusual. It was also the simplest and one of the most enjoyable. In 1975, Pope Paul VI decided to hold a Holy Year, when Catholics from all over the world would be encouraged to make a pilgrimage to Rome.

The Order of Malta were asked to provide first-aid and ambulance services in St Peter's Piazza and it was arranged that different national associations would accept responsibility for different months. The Irish being strong in the ambulance sector took on three months and I was invited to take charge of a team for two weeks. The Irish teams each consisted of twelve volunteers, all paying their own expenses, as is the rule in all the operations of the Order. A doctor accompanied each team. There was to be a short period of overlap, so that each group could brief its successors.

The previous team had my friend Frank King as doctor. He had been at Clongowes with me, in the same class and we were life-long friends and it was pleasant to see him again. Frank had ended up as Colonel in the RAMC, had retired, but still ran his show with military precision.

When we got to Rome, we were brought to a middling sort of hotel, where they were careful to put us in some kind of annexe. We then went along to establish contact with the Vatican. The Order had set up a clinic in one of the wings running out of St Peter's before they reach Bernini's colonnade. On the piazza side there was a fenced area, with our sign up and a throughway to an open area at the back where we had our ambulance.

Our lot were so good and so efficient that I was really hardly needed and I led from behind. It was exciting to see our team in action. The men were like sheep-dogs ranging through the huge crowds, up to 100,000 each evening. Perhaps a young nun would get excited and climb on a bench, only to fall off and break her ankle; before she knew what was happening she would be on a stretcher carried high above the crowd to our clinic, where we would do up her ankle in a temporary splint, then in the ambulance to the hospital, an x-ray and a plaster cast, to be followed up and taken care of later. Or, an elderly Dutchman and his wife, coming to Rome for the Holy Year to give thanks for her recovery from a cardiac ischaemic incident, would be horrified to see her blow up like a balloon with anaphylaxis from something she had eaten. He would sit crying, anticipating the bringing of her home in a coffin, only to see her return to normal in a few minutes after I had given her a shot of benadryl. To see that old pair go off with their arms around one another was a joy.

To crown the whole occasion, we were succeeded by a Lurgan team. They were headed by Dr MacCaffrey, looking like a picture in her uniform. The party had as captain, one Noel MacGrann, very dear to me, as I had brought him into the world and whose bottom I had smacked to make him take his first breath, one Christmas, long ago. He was something of a hero and had been decorated by the Order for bravery under fire with his Ambulance Unit in the troubles in the North of Ireland. I was delighted to see the Lurgan folk and for a couple of days, I became 'Dr Jim' again.

Tagoat

Life on the farm at Rathdowney was very good for us. For me it meant plenty of hard work on the tractor and in the care of the cattle. We followed the cycle of the growth of grass, cut and made silage, and wintered the cattle in yards. After a while I became a good stockman and altogether it was very pleasant. In Portmarnock, we had had a smaller acreage on our farm and went in for intensive land use, with a Jersey dairy herd, poultry and the growing of vegetables for the Dublin markets. This meant a lot of machinery and expense but we learnt and in Rathdowney we kept the whole thing simple.

I found Myles Mordaunt on the place, where he had been for nearly thirty years as working steward. I asked him to continue to work for me. He was an excellent stockman and a good gardener, but more important than that, he was the wittiest man I have ever known and one was guaranteed a good laugh every hour on the hour. When he retired, he was succeeded by Kevin Lynch, a complete all-rounder, having served in the Irish Army and then been a deep-sea sailor for many years. He has taken good care of us since.

My illusion of an old-fashioned farm, with ducks on the pond, hens pecking in the yard, butter being made and myself riding out on a sunny morning to survey the landscape, soon vanished. If I was not to go broke I had to get on the tractor and work hard the same as everybody else. Foolishness like ducks and hens and hunters soon vanished. But it became a bit lonely.

This was soon remedied when with some of my friends we set up the Tagoat Community Council. Tagoat is a small district lying between Rosslare harbour and Rosslare strand or Rosslare proper. The harbour is a small industrial complex of well-paid workers, tending the port. They have a railwaymen's club, a life of their own and there is always plenty going on. The Strand is a seaside resort, very genteel, with a beautiful beach, famous hotels, a good golf-links, a colony of retired people, well-heeled summer visitors, a good bridge club and plenty of entertainment.

Our area has about two hundred households, is small, has a few large farms, mostly owned by old people, some smaller farms, and a number of people who work at different things outside the district. There were a lot of pensioners and a horde of nice children. The district had an old corrugated-iron, disused school-house, which was the so-called parish hall.

We set up a Community Council and decided to build a modern community centre, and drew up a programme of activities. We had no money and the district was not rich. We divided up the work and each did what he or she knew best. My end was usually the paper-work and the negotiations with authority. Bit by bit, we gathered enough to get started. Then I negotiated an interest-free loan of £10,000 from Wexford Community Services Council as part of a revolving fund, which I proposed to them. AnCO used our project as a youth employment operation.

After some years of negotiations, I managed to secure from the Land Commission, a four acre field as a sports ground. Also in the package was an old derelict farmyard. When we examined this, we found that it was a very good example of a traditional mediaeval Yola homestead and was hundreds of years old. The Yola are descendants of a colony of West of England, Norman, Fleming and other folk, brought here about 800 years ago at the time of the Norman invasion and who survived and have kept their identity and language until present times. We are developing this as a folk centre to perpetuate their memory. We will use it for a cultural, and particularly, as a tourist centre of interest.

The Council has a programme for our old people. They are all visited each month and their problems noted and dealt with. All their houses have been put in good repair. For teenagers, we have weekly discos, handball and badminton and football teams. There is a fairly good programme of other activities. For the school children we provide school lunches at the Centre during the winter. Old people and others also attend for these meals.

We do quite a lot of case-work in personal and family problems and are trying to build up a career-guidance service. The
officers of the Council are always available for advice and
help. We have a very good Emergency Service; a fall of snow
brings out the young men on tractors and they go around
checking on the welfare of the old folk and bring them bottled
gas, bread, milk or whatever they might need. A small local
river was choked and flooded the lands of seventeen riparian
farmers. We organised a drainage scheme which has been successful. We bring deprived city children for holidays and a few
years ago, during the British coal strike, we had a group of
Welsh miners' children over for a visit.

The Community Council development has proceeded apace.
On the restoration of the Yola Farmyard we employ ten men
and are well on in the work. We have also begun a genealogical
project and are transferring all the material on the parish
records of the parishes in the two baronies of Forth and Bargy
on to computer memories and are also examining graveyard
tombstones, old newspaper references and so on with the idea
of providing information from this material for anyone with
Yola or other background from this area who may want information on his or her ancestry. We have another ten people
working on this including an archivist.

Then we have an office, which provides an infrastructure
and which is well-equipped with a computer and other items.
Ten youngsters are working there and they get work experience. We also run a laundry for old people, an office and
information service for the community, school meals and other
activities. Sixteen young people trained in this project have
been successful in securing jobs. One way or another, under
various schemes we are employing about thirty people, which
is not bad for a little community of 200 households. We have
had all kinds of adventures. For example, some years ago,
when the first Anti-Nuclear Rally was held at Carnsore, Pat
Stafford, my esteemed colleague and I went to see what it
was all about. It was raining very heavily and was pretty deso-
late and Pat, a Meteorological Officer forecast that it would
continue for the three-day Rally. We found that the organisers
had made no provision for food for the participants. So I got
out my tractor and hauled things about and within an hour

or so we had a canteen going, under scaffolding and tarpaulins and we fed the 7,000 people there, for three days. We had sixty of our people working, around the clock, and we sold thousands of loaves, sandwiches and so on. There was no rip off, ten pence for a mug of tea, coffee, or soup. We made a fair sum, which helped to pay for the Community Centre. This performance was repeated at the next two anti-nuclear rallies. I occupied my usual role: having started the show, Pat and my friends, much more able than me, took it over and made a 'go' of it by doing all the work.

I was living in a quiet, happy obscurity when one day, Dr John O'Connell, at that time Ceann Comhairle of the Dail, (The Speaker), also Editor of the *Irish Medical Times*, rang me and asked if he might send a journalist to interview me with the idea of doing a 'Profile' for the *Times*. Denis MacClean duly turned up and spent a while with me. It was Denis who insisted that I should write this book. Anyway I was written up in the *Irish Medical Times* under the caption of 'Portrait of a Genius' which was highly flattering, if a bit nonsensical.

To show the power of the Press, I came back from the 'shadows' and came under notice again and things began to happen. First, I was made an Honorary Fellow of the Faculty of Community Medicine of the Royal College of Physicians in Ireland. Then Queen's University of Belfast made me an Honorary Doctor of Science. This pleased me enormously since very few Public Health people ever receive such an honour. This kind of thing is usually reserved for academics and research people. I appreciated it even more because of my background in the North of Ireland and the generosity of spirit of the present-day Queen's Academic Authorities.

Then the Sovereign Military Order of Rhodes, Malta and Jerusalem (The Knights of Malta) made me a Grand Officer of Merit for work I did for them, years ago, on Leprosy. There were other things, but the most interesting was that, from more than two hundred people nominated by bodies engaged in community and social work all over Ireland, I was awarded the honour of National Pensioner of the Year. I was nominated by the Wexford Community Services Council. The Award was sponsored by the Irish Life Assurance Company and meant a handsome trophy and a generous gift for the Tagoat

Community Council. So it is wonderful what a press notice can start for someone!

For me all of this local community work in latter years has been wonderful in enabling me to know and enjoy my neighbours and to give me still something to think about and to provide a purpose in my life. I represented Tagoat on the Executive of the Wexford Community Services Council, an umbrella organisation for our area of Wexford town and the district, which has more than fifty affiliated voluntary bodies. But the most important thing, after the work we do for people, is the friends I have made. To be still of service and of use to the community at my age is pretty marvellous. Of course it has not been easy. Like all Irish enterprises we have the inevitable splits, have had rows, disagreements and even at times a certain amount of unhappiness and strain. But it has worked out well in the end and has been worth it.

Epilogue

I wrote several versions of an epilogue for this book, each trying to distil the wisdom and the lessons to be learnt from my sixty years of life since I first 'put up my plate' in Lurgan. However, by chance, something happened which is a fitting epilogue for my case-study of *To Cure and to Care*, so here it is.

A short time ago, my wife was in hospital and I decided to go to the Cistercian Monastery in Moone, Co. Kildare, there to spend a few quiet days. In the flurry of packing and finishing up various small tasks and fussing about, I overdid things and so suffered a mild 'heart-attack'. When the doctor came, he wasn't too happy at my progress and before I was aware of what was happening, there was an ambulance on the driveway and I was whisked off to hospital where I was installed in the acute medical ward, one down from Intensive Care. So that instead of one caring institution, the Cistercians, I found myself in another, the Hospital. When I had collected the various parts of my personality together again and found that I wasn't too bad and was not going to pass on just yet, I settled down to watch the scene in the ward and to relate it to this book.

The first recollection was an appreciation of the mixture of good high-technological medical care and the sheer down-right 'hands-on' excellent nursing to be seen in that ward. As a doctor myself, I won't say too much about the medical care. Because of the hospital staff's reputation I expected it to be first-class, which of course it was. The nursing was a perfect example of what I have been talking about all through this book. First there was the spirit and the atmosphere and the determination in that place. An old man in the next bed to me, aged well over eighty, who lived alone and had been found unconscious on the floor by his neighbours was so ill that I thought he would die during the night. But those caring nurses kept him going and worked on him to such an extent that a couple of days later they had him sitting out in a chair and feeding himself, from there he went on to a comfortable geriatric home. Second, I watched them come on duty in the morning, fresh and bright and saw them weary and worn after their day's work. Third, the caring and personal attention was an example of real devotion and dedication. Night and day the nurses were on patrol, unobtrusive but missing nothing and by sheer will and motivation and helping, inspiring the patient group in that ward to get better.

Lying there, I reflected that a hospital is simply a shell or an instrument in which skilled people work to provide a service and a hospital is only so good as the people who work there. The service is provided in relation to and to meet the needs of the community and an operation of closing beds really means reducing the service to the community. People talk about closing beds or hospitals. What they really are talking about is terminating services which sick people need.

I thought of the hospitals when I was a young doctor long ago in the North and the state of the wards and the care available and contrasted it with what I was experiencing. I thought of the years of work and development by so many people, which had been necessary to bring the services up to the standard which now exists. Of the training the nurses had received, the spirit which enthused that ward, of their dedication and how easy it would be for the daft social control which has now taken over, to turn the place into a shambles. I remember during the war when the excuse, 'There is a war on' was enough to allow laziness, idleness, apathy and low standards. I prayed that the work so many had put into building up this magnificent service should not suffer. I remembered that what is happening today is simply a continuation of the struggle between the penny-pinching Guardians and the doctors, who fought to get decent care for the poor, sick and hungry in the workhouses. I also thought with pride, that the things that we had inaugurated more than forty years ago had had a magnificent result and given a reasonable chance further improvements were certain.

This whole business of care is not the responsibility of

accountants, balancing the books or of economists allocating scarce resources or of the diktats of administrators or of politicians following ideologies, it is really the responsibility of the people delivering the care. Of those patients in the ward, some owed their survival to the prompt diagnosis and action of their family doctors, others were heart operation cases brought in for assessment, so that care extended widely before and after the admission of the people to that ward. It is a continuing care, something built up over decades, something wonderful to achieve and something which could be destroyed by commercialism, by bureaucracy or by political interference.

I remembered the man going down from Jerusalem to Jericho, who fell among robbers and was beaten up and was left half dead and the good Samaritan who rescued him while the priest and the levite passed him by. The Samaritan went to him, bound up his wounds, set him upon his own beast and brought him to an inn, where he gave the inn-keeper two denarii, saying 'Take care of him, and whatever more you spend, I will repay you when I come back'. Here is the Western world, never so rich, cutting down on its health services or trying to get them on the cheap and yet meanwhile earning enormous obscene sums, selling arms to the Third World to enable others to kill one another. What hypocrisy. However it is inevitable that people will demand that health care should be available as a human right, and that care be provided on a basis of need rather than on an ability to pay. This was the spirit in which the nations agreed to provide health as a human right when they signed the WHO Convention more than forty years ago.

When you are over eighty and in an acute ward in hospital it is conducive to thought. So I had a spell of reflection in which I was like a character in one of Beckett's plays, in such a work as *Malone Dies*. I thought, how funny it would be if Neutrino particles really turned out to be Angels and how surprised my nuclear friends in Cern in Geneva would be if Neutrinos lined up as a sort of Heavenly Choir. I wondered what made them fly around, the Neutrinos I mean, going right through the sun and coming out the other side and gallivanting all through Space? Were they on Heavenly Missions? I considered that if a scientist could believe in Neutrinos he could believe in anything. I wondered when I met the Lord, would

He apply Probability Statistics in assessing my credit or guilt? I wondered what the Lord thought of Popper's Rationality Principle? Having considered Heisenberg's Principle of Uncertainty, I was happy in my old-fashioned faith and belief in God and decided to hold on to this as being something which to me made sense and was really pretty wonderful. Then in my stream of consciousness, I thought how lucky I had been, with a wonderful wife and happiness for more than fifty years as well as the devoted family we have. How fortunate I had been in being able to do all the things I had wanted to do, or very nearly. How blessed I was with the wonderful life I had had, how silly so many of the periods of anguish seemed to have been, what wonderful friends I met and what fun my life had been. In that ward, there was a calmness and peace, jokes, and a friendly companionship among the eight men, there confronting their fate. When my blood pressure climbed up again from the pits and I was ready to leave, I was sorry to go. I had experienced what care, kindness and human goodness can give to an old body like me, in terms of Renewal, Faith and Hope.